Life Tried to Throw Me a Curveball:

I Overcame Diabetes to Become a Pro

Dave Caiazzo

with Paul Leahy

First published by Dog Ear Publishing
4010 W. 86th Street, Ste H
Indianapolis, IN 46268
www.dogearpublishing.net

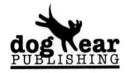

ISBN: 978-145750-681-9

This book is printed on acid-free paper.

Printed in the United States of America

Dedication

This book is dedicated to Angeline and Rocco, the best parents a son could have, and to Steve and Joan, the best brother and sister anyone could grow up with.

"The one constant through all the years is baseball."

– James Earl Jones as Terrence Mann in *Field of Dreams*

This is the story of one man's journey through life and how baseball has been interwoven through that life since his father handed his young son a baseball and glove. The physical journey has taken him from his hometown in Malden, Massachusetts, to New Haven, Connecticut, to Butte in Montana, to countless baseball parks from Massachusetts to California.

During the journey, he has met, been coached by, and played with and against a wide variety of singular characters, many of whom remain his friends today.

Preface

BACK IN THE YEAR 1964, the family got the scare of our lives when Rocco had a major heart attack. Two days before, we were playing our Sunday game of baseball at Amerige Park. I remember Dad hitting baseballs out of sight into the tennis courts a good distance away. He definitely was overexerting himself. We, back then, didn't think much of it because death wasn't thought of much when we were young. He was running around the bases and working himself pretty good. The next day we went to a Red Sox game and were walking from the car to the ballpark and Dad stopped and you could see he was losing and trying to catch his breath. I went back to him because he had stopped and asked him if he was alright. He said yes but also said for me to go ahead and he'd catch up. I was scared. Of course, I waited for him. I was only ten years old then. We finally made it into the game and everything seemed fine with Dad.

A day or so later was the day he had a major heart attack and was rushed to Mass. General Hospital in Boston. The doctors worked on him feverishly. Apparently, he had technically died for a short time but fortunately for everyone, especially our Caiazzo family, the doctors brought him back to life. That was around the same time that President John F. Kennedy was assassinated. I remember going into the Mass. General Hospital to visit Dad. Each visit was with tears in my eyes. Each visit was special just seeing Dad speaking and talking with Mom, Steve and Joan. Nobody deserved what Dad was dealing with but especially him. He was the greatest father anyone could ask for - always so proud of all of us. He was, himself, a proud, proud man. Each visit to the hospital would bring flashbacks to me of playing ball with him, going away on family trips, taking family pictures in Boston, things like that. Mom was very upset with what had happened to Dad. She would cry at times. I never wanted to see Mom cry.

The family relatives would stop by and always ask if we needed help with things. I remember Uncle Cliff and Aunt Dulcie (one of my favorite aunts and my father's younger sister) constantly there in case we needed anything. Even the neighbors were concerned. The Bishop family who lived next door was deeply affected. They had lost their father a couple of years earlier. Tommy and Ronny Bishop were always with us. They loved my father.

After a lot of care and a lot of praying, Dad was back with us not only leading us in life but showing the love for his family he always did.

The more you talk about family, the more you hear people say that the father is always closer to his daughter than his son or sons. Now that wasn't necessarily the case in our family but Dad did have a special love for sister Joan. She adored Dad. He was always looking after her. But, then again, we all were. She was the youngest of us all. I remember later on, guys would come by to go on a date with Joan and after the dates on many occasions Joan would say, "Why did you guys scare so and so away." We'd say, "What do you mean?" She would says the guys were intimidated by being greeted at the front door by two big brothers, over 6-foot, 3-inches tall. Joan later got into modeling for Barbizon Company. She didn't pursue it for long but Mom and Dad would always push her in that direction. She had the Caiazzo height and the Italian good looks. She was attractive to most everyone.

Right around this time with Dad recovering and beginning to get back into everyday life, we received another jolt to the family. Dad's father, Noni Nick, was found dead in Medford. It still is not known to this day what actually happened to him. He was found in the water in the Wellington area of Medford. Noni was a big, strapping, handsome man. He was a giant back in his day. He had a hand as large as a catcher's mitt. Noni Nick used to like to gamble a lot and the family doesn't know if he owed money to someone or if he was depressed over a family problem but now he was dead. I remember Dad was at work the day Mom got the word from the family. So when Dad came home, I remember sitting at the top of the stairs listening without being visible to what Mom was going to say to him. She told him and Dad took it like a man. Now Noni was gone but his memory was still with us.

I remember going over Noni Nick and Noni Matilda's house every Sunday. I still feel how painful it was to give Noni Nick a kiss on the cheek. He never was clean shaven and it was rough skin. He still had the old wine machine in his basement and would make his own wine. Those years were fun. All the cousins, aunts and uncles would go over to the house in Everett on Sundays and stay all day. Uncle Louie (Dad's oldest brother) would come by with his wife Aunt Lucy and cousin Nick, younger brother Lou and sisters Marie and Rita. Uncle Jerry (Dad's older brother) and his wife Amelia with son Jerry Cai and sister Linda. Then there was godmother Aunt Josie (Dad's sister) and her husband Tom Giannino (my godfather) and their children, Tommy, Bobby, Terri and Kevin. Kevin and I ended up playing semi-pro baseball for a few years. He was a good third baseman.

One of my father's closest family members was his sister Dulcie and her husband Uncle Cliff who was always the person who would help out with family matters. He was a great guy through the years. Aunt Dulcie and Uncle Cliff had two daughters Caroline and Janice along with brothers Lou DiSanto and Jimmy. Lou is the person nowadays who knows everything about the family. Growing up, he was a bit older so we weren't that close but now we are very close and he really shows a great interest in my past and what I did on the ball field. He's a wonderful guy who recently got married to his lovely wife Diane. My father's youngest brother Tony is still alive but recently lost his wife Aunt Betty. Their children are Richie, Kenny, Paul, Mary Jean and Elizabeth. Uncle Tony was almost a lookalike for my father. I look at his old driver's license and I'm amazed how much he resembles Dad. I often ask him to pull the ID out for me to look at my father again.

Many nights, due to Dad struggling with his work in Boston, we had to pinch quite a bit at the dinner table. Dad always put food on the table and a roof over our heads, but some nights were a little tough to take. Dad had a meal for us that I don't think any of us liked. He called it "La Zoup." It was bread soaked in a bowl of hot cocoa mix. That was supper. But that was one way of having dinner but not in an extravagant way. We would have that sometimes two nights in a row and maybe another once or twice a month. Dad and Mom were also great with taking us out to dinner at Anthony's Pier 4 or Jimmy's Harborside, two of the best restaurants in Boston at the time. Steve and I were dressed up in our suits and Joan in her little dress. We were only nine to twelve years old at the time so it was a big deal. And no other family in the neighborhood would do things like that. Mom and Dad always did it right for us.

1.

The Foundation, Both On And Off The Field

NOW WAS THE TIME I was starting organized baseball. My first team was the Redbirds but now was the Dodgers in the Malden Little League. I played well at nine years old against the ten-, eleven- and twelve-year-olds. The one thing I remember most was facing the best pitcher in the league, a kid named Rich Sylvestri who was a twelve-year-old. In that game, I pinch hit and in the last inning with us down by a run, I hit a long fly to center field and their centerfielder leaped over the fence to rob me of my first home run and also the game-winner. But at that point I knew I could play.

As an eleven-year-old, it was a big deal to be the starting pitcher on an all-star team but I was set to pitch in the game. However, because I was starting to play around with curve balls, I hurt my arm and couldn't pitch. I had to play first base. An umpire, Tony DiBennedetto, had taken a liking to me as a ballplayer and said he wanted to show me a curve ball. I always said why did I need to throw a curve? At that point, I was throwing fast balls by everyone. One game against the Braves I struck out every batter I faced in six innings. As of today, the kid I beat, Mike Gagliardi, still carries the article that was in the newspaper back then in his wallet to show me again.

I could see the progress each game, each year. By the time I was twelve, I was the number one pick coming out of the Little League and going into the Malden Babe Ruth League. I was chosen by the Colts. Those Little League years were fun but now the Babe Ruth League was next. There were some good ballplayers in the league but none that stood out. There was one kid in particular, Joe "Rocket" Ragusa. Everyone feared him and all I heard about him was as a pitcher. When I saw him and faced him, he did look good. One time I was facing him in junior high school and I beat him by 5-0. I bested him on the mound but once I faced him at the plate I didn't think he was that great, but he was good. In that game, I went three-out-of-three against him and knocked in four of the runs.

In 1968, I was going into junior high school (Beebe) where I now wanted to have people notice me. Those years were a little cloudy for me in terms of remembering much. I do remember my future high school baseball coach Frank Adorn being a teacher at Beebe. Tony Bavaro also taught at the school. Later in life I dated Tony's daughter, Robin. She was striking and always held big jobs with the state. I really liked Robin and she wasn't even born when I had Tony as a teacher. Mark Bavaro, the great tight end for the New York Giants and Philadelphia Eagles, was Tony's older son and David was the younger. He also played in the National Football League for a number of teams.

I considered myself at this time very naïve and was just starting to find out who I was as a person. It was getting close to baseball season and we were in gym class getting ready to change in the locker room when a kid came up to me to talk. His name was Bobby Harrison who we called Harry. He later was a teammate of mine at Malden High School. But this one day in junior high he came up to me and said, "I hear you're going out for the baseball team" I said, "That's correct." He said with a confident look on his face, "Do you think you're going to beat me out?" I kind of paused but then said, "Yes, of course I will." Harry turned out to be a good guy but he wasn't going to think I was taking a back seat to him. I can't remember much of Harry in junior high but in high school he did well. The one thing he did have was a strong arm.

That year we had a good team but not great. The next year, and the last before getting to the high school, was exceptional. I started to blossom. The coach was our gym teacher and he came to me one day and said, "You have a bright future ahead of you." That made me feel great and made me work even harder. The big game that year was when we played the Malden High junior varsity. They came to our park (Amerige) and in that game I hit two home runs completely out of the park. That was the biggest news around town. The next day in school, everyone was just yanking at me wherever I went. Then in history class as I entered the room, Tony Bavaro was looking at me. When we got inside the classroom, he said "I heard you had quite a game yesterday." Boy, did that make me feel great coming from him. Tony was quite an athlete playing for the San Francisco 49ers before an injury cut his career short. Tony and Frank Adorn were close so I knew Frank was not only getting word from Tony about the game but also from the JV coach, Bill McCormack, who also was a teacher at Beebe and good friend with Frank. So going into high school the next season was going to be exciting. I think I manufactured the script for what was to come.

My last year in Babe Ruth baseball at fifteen-years-old, I was chosen for the all-star team. At this time I had just completed my sophomore year in high school and I was one of the starting pitchers but also the starting shortstop. So one day we were practicing for all-stars and we were working on rundowns and I was at shortstop. We started the rundown and got the runner tagged out on one throw. Well, the manager at the time said, "Stop." He looked at me and said, "What are you doing?" I looked at him and said, "What do you mean?" He said, "We want you to wear this kid down by making as many throws as possible so he doesn't come back late in the game to hurt us with the long ball." That was a "can't believe you made that statement." I knew that we made the correct play. This is the type of thing you deal with in the early baseball years.

I was now getting myself geared up for high school baseball at Malden. As a sophomore, I showed Coach Adorn I could play. I pitched in about four games and played pretty well in the field. My brother Steve and a kid named Jim Coleman were the stars of the team my sophomore year. Jim was more of a contact hitter and a pretty good glove man and Steve was big and strong and could power the ball far and deep. They both pitched, as well. Jim was crafty and threw a lot of breaking balls and Steve threw hard. Sometimes he tried to overthrow. To this day I tease him about it. Brother Steve had a lot of talent but really was focusing on his football career. He always says to me he wishes he had my drive and determination. Steve went on to big time college football at the University of Minnesota in the Big Ten.

Just around this time my sophomore year in high school, I was going downtown to Malden Square each night hanging out with the other kids in school. Russ Hall was quickly becoming my best friend. He was a great guy. You could see how we had a lot in common right away. Russ played baseball but will be the first to tell you he wasn't that good but I give him more credit than he gives himself. He was a pitcher and played Babe Ruth League baseball, Legion and high school. One time Russ was pitching in a Legion game and was starting to get lit up and I was yelling in from the outfield to him for support. We always joked about that game and he used to say how I was intimidating him from the outfield. But he took it pretty good, although I didn't like to lose whether I was pitching or playing in the field. But he knew that's the way I was. When we were trying out for the Legion team, I came home from the practice and Russ came home with me. Steve asked us how we did and Russ said that he pitched and gave up a home run. Then Steve asked me how I did and I said, "I hit the home run." See. It didn't matter who I was competing against. I was out to win all the time; it didn't matter against whom.

Russ and I were always going down to the Square to hang out every night of the week. One thing besides meeting with the girls was going to Brigham's for hot fudge, strawberry or butterscotch sundaes. Each night we would do this. Then I started to feel myself getting thirsty quite often and craving sweets. It was going from one sundae a day to two or three. It was getting so bad I was now going behind the church in the Square to urinate. Each night was getting worse, not only going for the ice cream but now for milk shakes and frappes and sodas. Instead or urinating once a night, it was now seven or eight times.

One day I wanted a big steak and Mom made one for me to eat for supper but I could only look at it; I couldn't bring myself to eat it. I still craved sugar. During school hours I was leaving the classroom constantly to go to the bathroom. It was getting bad. I was starting to lose weight from urinating so much. This went on for quite a long time until one day I couldn't bring myself to go to school. I stayed home this one day and as soon as everyone in my house went to work and school , I walked down to the store and bought three half gallons of ice cream and two half gallons of milk and just made frappes and shakes all day long.

Later that day Steve came home from school with Doug "Superman" Balakovich and they said, "Let's go. We're bringing you to the hospital." They actually carried me and put me in the car. At the hospital, they diagnosed me with Type 1 diabetes. At the time I only knew one boy from the elementary school who had diabetes. The only thing I remember from him was he had reactions quite often and they had to give him sugar to raise his blood sugar level. I was in the hospital for about a week. The one thing I was concerned about was whether or not I could play baseball with this disease. I was told I could but had to keep a close watch on my blood levels. The doctors sent me to the Joslin Clinic in Boston to study up on the disease and learn how to give my insulin and learn what I could eat and couldn't. It was difficult. My mother had to take time off from her job at Gillette's to help to learn about diabetes.

The girl I really liked at the time was a girl named Karen who later was queen of the prom when we went together our senior year. When I was at the overnight area of the Joslin Clinic for a week, Karen organized about twenty-five people (classmates and friends) to come and visit me. That meant a lot. Later, Karen and I broke up but we had a good time. One time when we broke up, Karen dated a big basketball player from Malden named George. I was the jealous type and I didn't like being teased by the guys regarding that matter. After a while, I said to everyone that I'd take care of the situation. Well, one day we were in Malden Square again and George was in Brigham's and I waited for him. When he came out, I approached him and said "Let's take care of this situation now." I said "Let's go" and started to go to the back of the church. He knew I wasn't happy. He kept saying "Let's talk. Let's talk." I said "No!" We went behind the church and we squared off with everyone watching. I remember hitting him once and he went down. It was over right away. I felt much better but I blamed Karen more for what happened than George He ended up with the worst looking eye anyone had ever seen.

The diabetes was getting to be something I constantly had to deal with but I did the best with it. A short time later I got a cut on my leg and, due to not healing properly because of the disease, it broke out all over my leg and it was gross. It took a while to heal but it finally did. This is something I realized I was going to have to deal with for the rest of my life.

Dad was still bringing home fruits and vegetables, cold cuts, rolls, and Italian bread from Haymarket where they had (and still have) the old carts filled with those items. Dad would come home with bags and bags of food. His hands had deep marks in them from holding those heavy bags and carrying them back from Boston on the subway after work. Instead of attacking all the food as I did prior to the diabetes, I had to watch the amount of everything I ate.

The Joslin Clinic got me squared away but it was a grind every day. I remember the doctors and nurses telling me that I was going to be tired each day and I would have mood swings. They said it's not your fault, it's just part of the disease. I could be laughing, joking one minute then go into a serious mood the next. It was tough with the girlfriends I had and now understand what they had to go through, as well. Due to the diabetes, I had lost about twenty pounds. I was at 165 pounds and went to 145. But I put it back on in time. I was always lean with the athletic build. Russell used to say "you have that strong athletic body with not an ounce of fat on you."

Having the disease now was going to mean giving my shot each morning, then eat my three meals a day and snacks in between. It was like a full-time job. My Dad always used to say it meant I would be eating healthier and would probably live a longer life due to it. But I had my doubts. One night while out with a few friends down Malden Square, I had a few beers not thinking it would affect me but wow did it ever. The guys lost track of me behind the high school; I almost passed out. They helped me, though, and I said I'll never get drunk again. I really don't think I ever did again. It was starting to feel to me like it was a never ending battle. Sometimes I felt like I just couldn't win.

2.

Joe Pep Came Into My Life

BASEBALL WAS NOW A BIG part of my life; playing wiffle ball games one-on-one in the yard each day, maybe twenty games a day. Russ would come down, Superman, Steve and I. I'd pull out the lineups of every major league team and change teams so I could familiarize myself with their pitching motions and batting stances from watching games on TV. Now, though, I had just found out one day when we were at Noni's house in Everett through family that New York Yankees first baseman Joe Pepitone was related to us. Well, let me tell you. I instantly became a Yankees fan, and Joe Pepitone fan, as well. Those were the years when the Yankees were great; Mantle, Ford, Maris, Howard, Richardson, Kubek, Tresh and so many more. Mickey Mantle quickly became my idol. I followed his every at bat. Brother Steve, however, was a San Francisco Giant fan with his idol, Willie Mays. They had a tremendous team themselves with Willie McCovey, Orlando Cepeda, Juan Marichal, Jim Ray Hart, and Jack Sanford, among others. We had our days arguing and playing against each other in the yard being the Yankees and Giants. I did win most of the time. We still laugh about back then but that's the way it was supposed to be anyway – the Yanks win.

One of the biggest days of my life was when my Dad said let's go see the Sox play the Yankees at Fenway Park. I'll never forget it. Rocco, always thinking of us, brought me by the Red Sox dugout where the Sox players were warming up playing catch. The Yankees were taking batting practice. Dad and I got down behind the first row of seats and signaled over to Frank

Malzone, the Red Sox legendary third baseman. We asked him to get Joe Pepitone's attention. Frank looked over and said to Joe, "Hey crazyman, some people want to see you." Here he came. I was ready to jump out of my clothes. He came over and Dad introduced us and they talked about Joe's mother being a Caiazzo. When Joe shook my hand, I'll never forget how big he was and that what a thrill it was for me. All I remember doing while he was in front of me was look at that New York jersey and hat. Leave it to Dad. He never disappointed us.

A few years later, Dad and I went in again to see the Sox and Yanks play. I kept asking Dad if he would see if we could meet Joe again. He said yes. In those days, most of the time we could take Dad's Chevy Impala in to town and find a parking space. For some reason, though, this day, we were running late. By the time we got into the park it was getting close to game time. I remember being a little upset because I figured this time we won't see Joe. But Dad, noticing that I was sulking, made his way down to the Yankee dugout area and was standing there for a few minutes. All of a sudden, who comes out of the dugout to talk to Dad – Joe Pepitone. After conversing for a couple of minutes, Joe and Dad both looked up at me with Dad pointing to where I was sitting and gave me a wave. Even the people around us were saying Joe Pepitone's waving to you. Dad came through again. After the game, however, Dad explained what happened when he went down to the dugout. He had seen a Yankee player standing there not knowing who it was and asked him if he could get Joe. The player responded to Dad by saying, "What do I look like, your valet?" Boy, was Dad angry. He later thought it was Clete Boyer after looking at the team picture. Even if it was, I still liked Clete Boyer.

Mom and Dad would make a habit of it each summer to take us all to New York. We would stay in some of the better hotels and then make our way to Yankee Stadium. What a ballpark where all the greats and Yankee ghosts played. Ruth, Gehrig, DiMaggio, Mantle, Berra, etc. Mantle was still playing, though. Just getting out of the subway was a thrill. When you exited the train, you were looking right into Yankee Stadium. One time we went but the park was sold out. Somehow, Red Barber, the great Brooklyn announcer, was going into the bleacher area to do a show. He caught a glimpse of my mother and he got us all into the park. I think he liked Mom. Mickey hit two home runs that day against the Cleveland Indians and Joe Pep hit one, as well. Big Steve Hamilton came in to nail it down for the Yankees. I'll never forget, when you saw number seven (Mantle) come out of the dugout, you saw 'God.' That's how I felt about Mickey Mantle. He was not like some of today's players who don't act professionally on the field. After hitting a home run, he just acted like it was supposed to happen.

As a junior in high school, I was starting to get recognized. Schools like the University of Pennsylvania, Arizona State, Rollins College, University of Mississippi, UMass, and Brown University were in pursuit. I had just completed a very successful Legion season. It seemed to people that even when I didn't have my best stuff on the mound, I was still winning. I hated to lose! Now as a junior I had a pretty good year. My record was like 4-1 after winning about six games in Legion ball. At school, the kids were noticing, as were the teachers. After the high school season, it was time for Legion again. My dominance was starting to take center stage. Our team was good but not one of the better teams in the league. One game in Somerville against that strong team I pitched against the great basketball player Mike Fahey. He went on in basketball with the Washington Bullets. But people may not know he was quite a pitcher. He was a southpaw but he could pitch. I'll never forget this game. We went twelve innings and tied 0-0. This was the first of six shutouts in a row. What a roll to be on. Our shortstop, Gary Campsmith, would say each game, "Let's just get one run with Dave and we win."

Steve had just completed his only season in high school football and what a year it was. He set all kinds of records; made some of the greatest catches you would ever see. He made one-handed catches like it was normal. One game in particular, he slipped while running a pass pattern and fell on his back. His quarterback who grew up with us named Perry Verge, threw the pass and while on his back, Steve reached up with two hands and caught the ball. Billy Tighe (Steve's Malden High coach who retired in 2010 as the oldest high school football coach in the country) said at the time it was the greatest catch he'd ever seen. Steve was All-Scholastic that year and went on to play junior college football in Nebraska at Fairbury Junior College. What a year he ended up having. Offers after his second year were coming in from all the biggest football colleges in the country; schools like Nebraska (which was number one in the country under Bob Devaney), Ohio State, Purdue, Florida, Florida State, and Minnesota, among so many others.

I remember answering the telephone one night when Steve wasn't home. It was Lee Corso who was at Louisville at the time. I was speaking with him and he asked me if I'd be interested in going there with Steve. He offered me a baseball scholarship. I'm sure he looked into my ability but really he wanted to do anything possible to get my brother there. Steve ended up signing on with the Minnesota Golden Gophers of the Big Ten. Steve wasn't happy he signed with them after being told they would throw the football but they rarely did. He went about six-foot-three and 260 pounds. And what hands. You didn't want to meet him not being his friend.

An incident in Malden Square one night caught everyone's attention, including Dad's. Steve was in the Square minding his own business when my catcher in high school, Carl, was screwing around and a car pulled over. Carl and the guy, who was pretty big, started mouthing off to each other. Carl, who had a wise mouth, pointed out my brother Steve to the guy. The guy said something to Steve and Steve responded by saying, "Get back in your car." He came toward Steve and Steve used the guy's head to ram a tree in front of a church. The face of this person looked like someone took a bat to him for twenty minutes.

Later, after the guy left holding his head, a bigger guy came down looking for Steve. This was the brother. There was a Riley's Roast Beef in the Square back then with sharp rocks sticking out of the entrance. He came after Steve with a pipe, swinging it. He hit Steve in the elbow with it. Well, that was it. Steve went crazy and pulled the pipe out of his hand and scraped the guy's face up and down the front of Riley's. The next week someone saw the guy with his entire head bandaged up. Steve got arrested by the local police due to the incident but they let him go early the next morning. When he came home he still had to face Rocco. But Steve gave Dad some story how when the college hears about stuff like this they'll eat it up. Dad bought into it.

Now, Dad and Mom were facing the fact that their two sons were probably going in the direction of big time football and baseball. Rocco was bringing people such as cousin Nick Cai to the house, as he did when we were really young, to talk with us. Nick was a standout pitcher at Everett High years ago and signed with the Red Sox. Getting Nick out of bed was the difficult task for Dad. Nick liked to sleep late. He later went on to be an actor, actually trying to emulate what his uncle Rocco did in his Hollywood years. Nick went on to become Luke's security guard in the soap opera General Hospital and in a number of movies. Before Dad met Mom, while she was still Angelina Colantonio, he was a model in New York and while at a party with some big people, someone approached Dad and said what you read about. An agent came to him and said, "I can make you a star." Rocco was amazing. While in Hollywood he dated actor Gary Cooper's future wife. Dad was asked to audition to be Rudolph Valentino in the movie "The Life of Rudolph Valentino."

When you saw Rocco's scrapbook and many pictures in his younger years, he was better looking than any actor you would see. Dad was much like me in that he didn't drink. Also, he was pretty straight. Although he had many women before falling in love with Mom, he didn't abuse himself. But Rocco declined the movie and soon returned home. He really wasn't sold on Hollywood in those days. Growing up, I used to talk to him constantly about that. Years later, a pretty good pitcher himself who I pitched with and who also was in the Angels farm system told me, "My mother and her friends say your father was the handsomest man alive. "

People seemed to think Steve and I got our athletic talents from our father's side of the family but my mother's side, the Colantonios, were talented, as well. As a matter of fact, my grandfather, Joe Colantonio, fought for the New England championship as a middleweight. He went by the name Joe Collins. I vaguely remember him because he died at a very young age. My mother always said he died from getting hit in the head so much. Those fighters take a beating. Mom's brother, Dom, also fought a little, as well. People from the North End of Boston, where the family grew up, still remember him as a fighter. My mother's other brother was Uncle Joe Jr., who loved to fly planes. He was a very quiet but interesting man.

My Aunt Thelma, who passed away recently, and Aunt Camila, the youngest sister, were always at our house when we were growing up. Cousin John and Tony Chiriciello (sons of Aunt Thelma and Uncle Tony) were always playing ball with us when visiting each other growing up. Mom loved all her brothers and sisters but had a soft spot for her youngest sister, Carol, who married Uncle Al Trifone. Al Trifone Jr. always stays in touch and is married to Liz. We all stay pretty close especially since Carol and Al and Thelma and Tony have passed on. Other than my Mom and younger sister Carmela, everyone has passed on Mom's side. Uncle Dom and Uncle Al have been gone for a number of years now. Michael Chrirciello (John's son) played a little college ball at UMass Boston. Growing up, you could see sister Joan was a good athlete, as well. She'd play in the yard, at times. My father would throw and hit ground balls to her and she'd handle it pretty well.

3.

Under The Watchful Eye Of The Red Sox at Fenway

DURING THE SUMMER OF MY junior year, the annual popular Hearst Record-American Sandlot All-Star Game tryouts were being held. They had about five or six dates and you had to showcase your talents in front of the Red Sox brass in Massachusetts and New Hampshire parks. I had pitched unexpectedly one night and the tryout I was planning to attend was the next day in Framingham. I pitched nine innings that day and went to the tryout the next day anyway. Frank Malzone was in charge and when I took the mound to pitch for them to about four or five hitters, he started to talk to me. I was throwing the ball by everyone but my arm was sore. Malzone leaned over to me and asked me if I had pitched the day before and I said yes. He responded with a "I know." He said he followed me. Then he said to just throw two more pitches and get off the mound. He said. "You made it." I'm glad he cut me short because it was hot that day and I was getting drained pretty much. I remember getting some juice I brought with me and guzzled down a couple of cans. My blood sugar must have been forty. But I was throwing on adrenaline.

My summer was now winding down. The big thing now was Fenway Park. I had just completed a great high school year where Frank Adorn gave me the MVP award at the sports banquet and my Legion season was getting close to the end and that was a huge success. A few days before the Fenway Park game I was pitching against Revere and struck out fourteen in six innings but hurt my back. Now I thought "How am I going to pitch?" Back in those days, Mayo Kaan was a famous chiropractor in Winthrop. (Kaan was a former bodybuilder who claimed to be a model for television's Super-man.) Someone recommended that I go see him so I made an appointment. He asked me some questions and then told me to look to my right. When I did, he snapped my head to the left. I felt nauseous but it helped. There was no way I was not pitching at Fenway Park. I think I hurt my back by emu-lating Juan Marichal. That was one fault I had as a kid. I watch so many players I liked so I would copy their delivery or batting stance but this time it cost me. The relatives were all at Fenway including my family and Uncle Jerry who was so proud of anyone in the family who excelled in sports. Coach Frank Adorn also was in the stands.

The diabetes was not causing me any problems up to this point and I felt pretty good but the back was still bothering me a little. When I got to Fenway Park, I was just in awe of the yard. Johnny Pesky, the legend who I became friends with later in years, had a bunch of the kids in the outfield. He said, "Fellas, as far as I'm concerned, Ted Williams shits ice cream." He loved Ted Williams By the time I got into the game, I was about the fifth pitcher of the day. I got to the mound and never psyched myself out by look-ing at the famous wall. I faced six of the top hitters in the state and put them all down. I never threw the ball as hard as normal but I was pitching and got everyone out. From that experience, I was ready for the next step up. Peo-ple now heard about what the Red Sox thought of me and what people saw of me against good competition. From that, expectations were rising. Scouts from major league teams were now starting to pursue me along with colleges from around the country.

Everyone was starting to get excited about the future. The Caiazzo family was starting to grow up now but Dad's business as a barber in Boston was starting to slow down dramatically. The South Station building where my father's shop was located was due to be torn down because of renovations. Mom was still working, as well, but things were getting tight. Good thing that Steve was getting a full scholarship now from the Univer-sity of Minnesota for football. That helped tremendously. I don't know how people can pay for college expenses for their children, especially nowadays. But everything is relative. My Mom and Dad never really deprived their kids of anything. If we needed a new baseball glove or bat or cleats, we got it. And it was the very best equipment. However, when things were getting tough, they would put their foot down. I remember when things were bad if we couldn't afford to buy much food, my father would say we're having La Zoup for the next couple of nights. That was chocolate milk or cocoa warmed up with a slice of white bread soaked in the chocolate milk. We tol-erated it. The other thing Dad would do is: if we abused the telephone situ-ation and built up the phone bill too high, he would put a small lock on it for a few days so we would learn not to spend a lot of time on it or make too many calls building up the monthly cost. We would get mad but Dad was the boss. But anything to help our careers, etc., he would do. He also had me take professional golf lessons at Franklin Park Golf Course. I did it for a while but said "no more!" The instructor said I could hit the ball a mile but I still wasn't going to do anything I wasn't happy doing.

4.

Women Were Starting To Catch My Eye

IT WAS THE SUMMER OF 1971 and the girls were really starting to catch my eye. Although I never had a problem getting women, it was trying to stay with one. To this day, I find myself losing interest very quickly. That has been a trait of the Caiazzos over the years. Dad didn't marry Mom until he was about thirty years old, and Steve later married around the same age. Being around a beautiful girl was so important to me. There was a girl I was starting to get close with around this time and she was very attractive but she had this minor little birthmark on her face and because of it I broke off with her. Every one of my friends were saying I was nuts but that was me. The girl, Linda, several years later ended up marrying a guy I graduated with.

My high school catcher, Carl, was starting to hang out with my group of friends pretty regularly now. Carl was basically a good kid but he had some major issues. He loved to drink and when he did, he was trouble. When you sat down with him when he was sober, he was a funny, personable kid but, boy, could he cause problems when you went out at night with him. Carl was pretty popular with the women but once they got wind of his act, it was "bye." Carl got me aggravated so much one time, we ended up play fighting. Nothing serious but I had him in a headlock and went to punch him in his stomach but I accidently hit his elbow and damaged the thumb on my throwing hand. To this day it is twice the size of my other one. It bothered me for quite some time.

We'd go out to nightclubs or bars and almost always end up having to break up a fight involving him. One time, outside of former Red Sox great Tony Conigliaro's nightclub, Carl was in a huge fight where we ended up coming to his aid. He could handle himself for not a big guy, though. A year or two after we got out of school, I had to confront Carl on some things. He was throwing my and Steve's name around like he would his own family. People were telling me about it. Finally, at Revere Beach, I grabbed him by the neck and picked him up and told him to stay away from me and Steve and I'd better not hear another word come out of his mouth regarding us. He got the message.

Even though the summer was winding down, we'd still be going to Amerige Park or Pine Banks Park to practice or play some pickup games. Sometimes I'd be the only one, throwing balls to myself or going to the front of our house on Rockland Avenue and throwing balls off the wall. I'd work on fielding backhands or going to my left on balls hit right at me. Karen was starting to take center stage with me. I had met her through Mom, who used to work with Karen's grandmother at Kennedy's Clothing Store in Boston. I was really beginning to like Karen a lot. She had this great body that I watched with giant eyes. She was a cheerleader, as well. But sometimes she took that too seriously. I mean, in those days, where were you going as a high school cheerleader? It wasn't like today where you go in pro cheering or open a dance studio or something. Many times we argued on that subject. There was always one of the guys in school trying to put a move on her and it annoyed me. There was this one kid, Peter, who basically was like a comedian but needed the attention. Karen knew he aggravated me. I used to tell her to stop talking to him when I was around.

The next year in high school I finally had an opportunity to get back at him. We would have street hockey games in gym class in the small gym. My team was playing against his team. I told everyone I want to go out on the floor when he's out there. He was a player on the varsity hockey team but that didn't mean a thing to me. When I saw him go out with his line, I jumped out to play against him. He was a bit overweight and was throwing his weight around checking smaller guys into the boards. Well, I waited until he got close and he tried to throw his weight at me and I maneuvered out of his direction and nailed him lifting him up off the floor. He hit the floor like a ton of bricks. That's all I wanted to do.

There was a girl who used to make me melt. She was in my typing class and her name was Wanda. She was the most beautiful girl in our class. I later played in the same outfield in high school with her brother Tony. Also, when my brother, Steve, was in Nebraska at junior college, Tony went there the next season. He was a pretty good football player. But I was really into Wanda. Tony used to tease me about fixing me up with her. I wish I had taken her out. Later on, years after high school, she became a Playboy bunny in California. That didn't surprise me, but she was a nice girl besides the looks and class she illustrated. Years later, we became very good friends and on vacations to California, I would see her but she was happily married.

5.

Twenty Ks In Eight Innings

STEVE WAS GETTING READY TO return to Fairbury Junior College for his sophomore year. I was going down to Pearl Street football stadium at night to throw him passes and work out. I'd be going back to the Joslin Clinic for my routine checkups and they would ask me how many times a day I was checking my blood sugar. I would tell them once or twice a day but to be honest I never checked my sugar once in thirty years. No lie. That was dangerous because I never adjusted my insulin to my blood readings.

One of my big things is, if you're going to say you're going to do something, make sure you do it. So many people make fools of themselves by not living up to what predictions they make. The sportswriters in the area used to like to talk with me before a big game and see what I would say. I tried not to ever disappoint; never give anyone reason to hold anything over you. I could feel myself dragging at times now that it was a couple of years since I got the diabetes. Waking up in the morning always was a challenge. People still didn't know much about the disease so I was really getting to understand it by feeling it. I was constantly tired. Never did a day go by where I felt good for most of the day, never mind all day. I really had to motivate myself.

Now the baseball season for my senior year in high school was upon us. Steve had just completed another football season and it was a great one. I knew I had a major handicap and knew I had to deal with it. You can't beat it but you can contain it the best you can. The Cincinnati Reds had contacted me regarding a tryout for them in Manchester, New Hampshire. I remember not feeling that strong that morning when I woke up. I tried to eat a little more than usual to keep me going but I still felt weak by the time I got to Manchester. By the time I got onto the mound to pitch, it was more physical than mental. The catcher was giving me signs and I couldn't even see them clearly. I must have crossed him up six or seven times. Someone can get hurt like that. The one thing I had going for me that day was that I was throwing hard. No one hit me. Cincinnati officials spoke with me afterward and said they were going to follow me closely the next couple of years. The diabetes was really acting up on me this day. When I got into the car to drive home, I passed out. Good thing I wasn't driving.

The funny thing about the tryout was that my high school catcher, Carl, was there and I faced him. I don't think he ever saw a pitch. He swung and missed at about ten consecutive fastballs and they told him to sit down. What a highlight film Carl was. The shame of it was that he was a pretty good athlete. Recently I came across John Romboli, a great athlete from Everett and a friend of mine. John caught me at Fenway Park and also was on the Everett team when I struck out twenty batters in eight innings. John told me he never let me know this over the years but when John came to the plate to face me in that game, Carl would say to John, "If you tell me what Luongo's throwing, I'll tell you what Caiazzo's throwing." He said he knew every pitch that I threw to him but said, "I still couldn't hit you." I threw some gas past John three or four times that game. I'm proud of that because he, and Frank Nuzzo and Johnny Capra were outstanding hitters. I couldn't believe when I heard what Carl was saying to them.

My senior year was just beginning and it wouldn't be long before baseball would be upon us. During the winter, I was in contact with many baseball universities around the country. I was drifting away from some of the kids I grew up with. We didn't have the same interests any more. One kid, Danny McDonald, I had known since we were about six years old. He eventually overdosed and died. He was a pretty good kid but let the wrong people come into his life. Ronnie Bishop ended up moving to New Hampshire. They were some of the friends of my early years.

The Yankees were no longer the real Yankees any more. The Mick had retired as did Whitey Ford, Elston Howard, Clete Boyer, and Bobby Richardson, Tom Tresh was now with Detroit, I think, and Joe Pep was with Houston or San Diego by now.

The Malden High School season had just begun. We were expected to be fair. As it turned out, our pitching carried us thanks to a young kid named Buddy Demontier. Buddy was just a great kid. He would ask my advice on pitching all the time. He had a very good arm. People expected me to be good but we did not know about Buddy. We opened the season at home against Somerville High School and I went the full nine innings striking out fourteen and winning 2-1. Buddy pitched next and won; he looked good.

At practice the next day, Coach Adorn told us he was going to scout Everett against Medford because Everett was our next opponent. We travelled to Everett by the usual bus. Mr. Adorn gave me the scouting report and told me to look it over. I never looked at that report. I knew they were a great hitting team. I said I was going to pitch to my strength, not their weakness. The opposing pitcher was Ron Luongo, a hard-throwing righthander. Years later, Ron became a close friend of mine. Ron could throw. We were in a great game when once again catcher Carl messed up a first-and-third situation and threw the ball into center field, not once but twice, scoring the two runs and we lost 2-1.

Ron Luongo struck out sixteen in nine innings and I struck out twenty in eight innings. Some major league scouts called it the best high school game they ever saw. But we lost and that's all I cared about. I didn't take losing too well. Luongo ended up signing a few years later, the same year I did with the Yankees. I never thought I struck out that many hitters in that game. What a crowd was watching, as well. That was a very draining game. I brought three cans of orange juice to that game and tried to spread them out. I really had no problems with the diabetes this day. Our team hitting was atrocious. So we knew as a team we had to get good pitching. For a sophomore, Buddy was outstanding. Russ used to say to me that everyone was expecting me to perform well and anything Buddy could give us was a plus. As I said, he gave us much more than that.

As the season went along, I think Coach Adorn was expecting us to be in the league race until the end. The major league scouts were starting to come around each game I pitched. Neil Mahoney, the Red Sox big guy in the scouting department, was there to see me beat Quincy 6-1. I started out shaky and a few other scouts left but Neil Mahoney and Tommy McDonald both stuck around to see me strike out fourteen and win my own game with three hits, including a three-run homer. After the game, I picked up Karen from work and we spent the better part of the night together.

Buddy beat Somerville the next game and then someone else pitched after that and we lost. Revere was another tough opponent but I got the ball that day and we won again. It was now getting to be fun. The night before that game I went down to Malden Square just for a short time and was going to call it an early night but some time during sitting on the church stairs, I got really low with my blood sugar. I went to the drug store to get some orange juice but I really didn't feel good the rest of the night. I was a bit worried about how I was going to get through the game but I did. I must have gotten only two hours sleep due to being low.

We faced Medford after that but we got belted. They beat us like 20-3. We threw a lefthander and another kid but it was a one-sided affair. Buddy pitched against Everett at our park but didn't have his usual stuff and we lost. I played left field and remember Frank Nuzzo hitting a ball to the left of me but well over my head for a tremendous home run.

The season was winding down. We faced Medford who was still in the race. The park where Medford played was a place I never liked pitching at. The night before I kept trying to say "forget about the park or the mound and pitch like I'm capable." Well, we beat Medford and I struck out the side in the ninth and ended up with thirteen strikeouts. Also, I hit a triple and single to knock in four runs. We ended the season in a three-way tie for first place but lost in the playoffs. I wasn't happy because I lost that game but it was the way I pitched that got me mad. My arm was really sore that game but I always said even with a sore arm I should beat anyone I faced. But I walked five or six hitters and hit two batters, as well.

After the season, the newspaper read "A tale of two arms." That pretty much summed it up. The team batting average was .189! I led the team in batting at .335 and the next hitter was Carl at .250. I was very proud to receive the MVP award at the school awards presentations for the second year in a row. At the event, we presented Coach Frank Adorn with a beautiful clock and pen and pencil inscribed plaque. He did a great job and was a coach you wanted to play hard for.

6.

Steve Ring Showing Me The Way

THE SUMMER SEASON WAS HERE and I had a big decision to make. Steve Ring was helping Coach Adorn part-time with the high school and was managing the semi-pro baseball team in Malden. He was rebuilding the team from the old Malden Mets. They were now the Malden Merchants. Steve had just got back from playing professionally with the Detroit Tigers organization. He took a liking to me and asked me to play for his team regularly. The year before I played in a few games for him, as well, but not many; I was only sixteen years old that year. So, was I going to play for the American Legion team or the Merchants? I decided to play regularly for the Legion team because I loved to hit and when Steve asked me to pitch, I would pitch for him. There were a lot of ex-pros in the Intercity League and it would help my confidence, etc., if I did well. Pitching my first game for Steve, I did well. The second time around, I got hit pretty well by a Lynnfield team that had some ex-pros in the lineup. I remember that due to rain-outs, I had a long layoff. During the game, I felt that I didn't have my good stuff.

After I lost that game, I learned an awful lot about myself and my arm. As I always did the next day at our game, I asked the catcher to catch me on the sidelines so I could work on my mechanics and pitches. Back then, you didn't have many guys who could help you much. While throwing on the side, my catcher said, "Wow, are you throwing tonight. Why didn't you throw like this last night?" Well, I said maybe I should throw more often and I got into a routine of throwing about five or six minutes the day before my next start. I found it livened up my arm. It worked. I was starting to throw great even though I was playing up in talent.

My catcher, Billy Ryan, who caught former Oriole Mike Flanagan at UMass, said I had a great fastball. He said "just keep everything downstairs." When he caught me, he stressed that; always pitching to a location. Billy was good for me. I learned an awful lot from him. I remember working one day on the sidelines with another teammate, Steve Shea, who just got released and was involved in the Rusty Staub-Donn Clendenon trade. Steve used to work with me on my curveball and started to help me throw a slider. The team ended up winning the league championship that summer after finishing fourth during the regular season. I pitched very well and Steve got me playing time in the field, as well. Steve got hurt in the playoffs and I had to fill in for him in left field. I saved one game with a catch going over my left shoulder. So the summer was a great learning experience between playing and just talking with the older guys. Steve Ring used to take me out to dinner and talk baseball with me all the time. He told me he believed in me and that I had a bright future. He was and still is a dear friend. Always concerned with my diabetes and if I was having any problems with it during a game.

7.

"I Thought I Was Going To Sleep With Dave!"

AFTER THE SEASON, IT WAS just doing my own work on the sidelines with Russ or my brother Steve and going out to the nightclubs almost every night of the week. One night, Russ, Carl and I went up to Sweeney's Roaring 90s in Rowley. We all met a girl that night. They all went to school at Northeastern University. They invited us over to the dorms. We told them we would meet them there later. We first had to get permission from Carl's parents to stay out late because they were watching Carl's every move now. They wouldn't let him go. So Russ and I went. When we got there, the girl I liked, a gorgeous brunette with a body you see in the magazines, was waiting for me. But the girl Russ was supposed to hook up with, I guess had her eyes on me. Before we were going to split up, the girls were talking, one saying. "I'm going to sleep with Dave." Then the other said, "I thought I was sleeping with Dave." This was going on for ten minutes. Russ, seeing this going on, kind of made a joke of it with his good nature. Everyone was happy at the end but to this day Russ still jokes about it to me. We had some fun.

Russ had his own women during those times, I just lucked out this time. Russ was always a good-looking kid. It's not like I was making fun of him as if he was a weird-looking character like some kids were. But we were best of friends and we could do that to each other and joke about it. We stayed over at the dorm but when I got up in the morning, I was really exhausted and needed to eat and take my insulin. Russ and I (especially Russ) loved the disco music so we started to frequent the discos. What great music and women!

I came to my decision on schools and instead of going to a large university, I came to the decision that junior college would be best for me. Mass. Bay Community College in Waltham was my choice. Mo Maloney had come to see me pitch a few times and was extremely aggressive in pursuing me. As soon as I got there, we began fall baseball. Fall baseball was only in its second year, and a few years later I ended up playing for the man who was the first to start it. During practices, Mo had Bill Monbouquette, former Red Sox great, working with me. I had a great fall, winning all my games and I batted fourth in the lineup hitting very well. Our team looked very good and was a big step from high school. We had D.J. Saulnier, a left-hander from Newton who had been drafted in the most recent draft by the Oakland A's. He was tough, and a good kid, as well. Mike Ryan was our catcher from the Braintree state championship team and John Greely was a good-hitting first baseman from Melrose. Jimmy Corrigan, a lefthanded-hitting outfielder from Medford, also was on the team. When the fall ended, we all had high expectations for the spring, and so did Coach Maloney.

Karen was now going to our Mass. Bay rival, North Shore Community College, and we had drifted apart by now. We would run into one another at times in the clubs but we didn't have much in common. I was starting to date a girl from Mass. Bay. Her name was Judy. She was a cheerleader for the basketball team. She was attractive and was from Sudbury. She came from money. When my father met her, he used to quiz Russ on her a lot. So I knew he liked her. My father still had great taste in women. I do recall that my catcher, Mike Ryan, really liked Judy and was in pursuit of her. When I would ask her about Mike, she used to tell me she had no feelings for him but that he was always calling her. One night after Judy asked me to pick her up at the Natick Mall, I got there a few minutes late. When I went to the mall, it was closed but I noticed some cars still in the parking lot. I saw what looked to be Judy's car and was looking inside to see if there was something I would recognize of hers. I even went to the other side of the car to look in since it was pretty dark. I recognized it as her car so when I walked away a few steps, I got a huge surprise. Mike Ryan's car was next to it and Judy was in the passenger seat. Judy gave me this look like "I didn't know he was going to show up" I talked to them and told them I was just in the area and figured I would see if Judy was working but I was embarrassed. Mike had a way of doing stuff like that, but he was a good kid, though. I just wasn't going to share my women with anyone.

The season was just about to begin. We started out great. We worked hard and we went to Cape Cod for our spring training back in those days. One incident in particular got everyone's attention. Back in those days, I was very private about my diabetes and didn't tell anyone except my coaches. Coach Maloney told me years later of how he was driving one day when we had an off day. When he was either going to or coming from lunch. He saw our leftfielder, Jim Corrigan, thumbing a ride with all his luggage. When Mo pulled over he said, "Where are you going?" Jim got in Mo's car and told him he was going home because there are players on the team doing drugs. Mo couldn't believe it and asked Jim what happened. He said he saw someone in particular shooting up with a needle in his arm. Despite being asked a number of times to tell him who, Jim wouldn't say who it was. Mo finally said, "Was it Dave Caiazzo?" Jim relayed, "Did you see him too, coach." Coach Mo smiled a bit and said, "No. Dave's got sugar diabetes and needs to take his medication every day." Jim was relieved and Mo brought him back to our motel in Hyannis. Mo said, "Caiazzo doesn't even drink a beer most of the time, he's certainly not going to take drugs."

The season was a huge success, individually and as a team. The game, of course, that I was looking forward to the most was against North Shore CC. When I ran into Karen, she would tell me what a great team they were going to have. Well, we faced them at the end of our season and John Tudor was their best pitcher. He went on to pitch for the Red Sox and Cardinals. But all I heard about was him. I said no way am I going to lose this game. We faced each other and our team won pretty handily. It was like 7-0. My season was pretty complete after that win. We took over sole possession of first place, went to the state tournament and won. I ended up 7-0 and was really throwing hard. My ERA was 0.45.

8.

Beginning The Greatest Dynasty In Intercity League History

NOW THE SUMMER WAS COMING and I was ready for Steve Ring's Augustine's Athletics team (He had changed the sponsor.). In the three or so pre-season games we played, I was throwing BBs, developing my other pitches, as well, and now perfecting that slider. We picked up guys like Ron Beaurivage from UMass and he later went with the Oakland A's; Charlie Meeker, previously with the Red Sox; and a kid named Joe DiSarcina, just back from the San Diego Padres and UMass. Boy, could he play shortstop. He made plays you've never seen before. Bobby Guidi, our shortstop the year before, was now playing second base. He was getting older so his days were winding down. A big plus was picking up Bob Corcoran, formerly of the St. Louis Cardinals, and a Yale righthander. He threw extremely well and what a class guy. The previous year we were starting our run and now it looked like we were going to keep up the pace.

Our main rival through these years coming up were the Joe O'Donnell-led Hosmer Chiefs. They had a long run at Intercity League championships but we were ready to end their run and pick up where we left off last year. They had some great players, Bob DeFelice (Red Sox), catcher; Ed Ride-out (former Patriot and Boston College receiver), a great shortstop; Dave Polcari, who I played with the year before and an ex-St. Louis Cardinal; Jeff Williamson, a righty who was just back from the Baltimore Orioles who was as good as they get; Ron Luongo, my opponent at Everett High who was also pitching well; and Mac McLaughlin, a lefthanded pitcher once with the Minnesota Twins. But we had our big boys, and were they big.

No one had to coach me into playing hard. It was in my blood. My future coach once said, "Dave is the nicest guy you ever want to meet but put him between those lines, he's as fierce a competitor you don't want to meet."

My brother Steve was now home for the summer from school and he was playing for us, as well. Steve had tremendous power and showed it throughout the course of that summer. People were amazed at the distances of some of his home runs. But Steve knew his future was in football.

Trixie (John Trischitta) was a very good friend of mine now and he had left Steve Ring the previous year because of a disagreement they had. Trixie was now with the Hosmer Chiefs. We played some games back in those years when the parks were packed. People would bring their chairs and fill them around the park, and fill the stands, as well. Trixie and I were always having friendly arguments and discussions about who was better, the Hosmer Chiefs or Augustine's Athletics. They were great years. Our uniforms were just like the World Series champion Oakland A's in those years.

Jeff Williamson and I were the aces of our staffs and when we faced each other the park was filled to the max. One game in particular, I pitched at home against them and it was written up pretty good. The sports writer called me early in the morning and asked me basically how the game was going to turn out that night. With my cockiness, I responded, "We will win tonight," and what a game it was. We won 2-1. As I've always said, I don't mind people "talking" if they back it up but if you can't back it up, I don't want to hear you, period. So I had to produce, and did. Williamson pitched great but it was a game both teams wanted badly. After the game, I remember Joe O'Donnell saying to me, "That was the best slider I've ever seen." That was a great compliment coming from Joe. He was a great athlete and was one of the greats in the league for some time. Joe's just a class individual.

Back in those days, the crowds were tremendous. I remember sometimes you couldn't even find someone you were looking for. By contrast, going to the games in the '90s and early 2000s, you could find who you were looking for right away.

Harry Mehos was our scorekeeper all through high school and he was with the Merchants and now the A's. I would drive him to all the games. He was just a great guy. He was fun to be with. Harry wasn't an athlete but he loved sports and really followed it. If we lost, Harry took the loss just as badly as we would. The A's-Hosmer rivalry was big to Harry. He would tell you things he heard one of the Chiefs say and want revenge. But I would always comfort him when I was pitching by saying, "Harry, we'll win and that's it." After a number of years, Harry believed everything I was saying. This was the beginning of the greatest dynasty in Intercity League history.

No one had to tell me that the next couple of years were very important to me if I was going to get drafted or sign as a free agent. Even though I wasn't signed out of high school, I knew I still had a few years to achieve that goal. Coach Adorn told me he used to discourage the scouts on trying to sign me because he wanted me to go to school so I figured that had to have a little something to do with it.

Vida Blue of the Oakland A's was the biggest thing in baseball at this time. What he started to do was run in and out from the dugout to the mound. I liked that and I began to do it. It was something else that might catch the eye of the scouts.

Before heading back to school for my final year at Mass. Bay, I was starting to see a neighbor of mine. Once again, the name was Karyn (spelled differently). She was an eye-catcher. I noticed her every day I'd be in the kitchen sitting down. She would park her Volkswagen in eyes-view of me. She always wore these revealing clothes. I said I had to look into this. One day I was outside when she was coming home from work so I waved to her. That broke the ice and we somehow started communicating. She was a good girl and also had an attractive older sister. We really didn't actually date for some time. One day I was talking to this girl I was interested in when she pulled her car over to talk. Well, Karyn was leaving her house and rode by and must have gotten jealous. The next day there was a note on my car from her asking who the girl was. Shortly after that we started dating. I would go over her house every night. She was great in bed but after a while it got old and I started to drift away. Just about the time I was ready to go back to school, she bought me a beautiful spiritual chain but I remember breaking it off with her but still wore the chain. But a year or so later, I lost the chain somewhere playing baseball. We dated a year later again but it wasn't the same. A few times while sleeping with Karyn I would either fall asleep on her or not be able to satisfy her. My diabetes was acting up, on me a lot at this time. I would get embarrassed but would always use the excuse that I was extremely tired lately from playing ball every day. I don't think she bought it, though. The diabetes was really starting to take its toll on me physically as well as mentally now.

School started at Mass. Bay. Russ was attending the Bay again for his second year. Russ was on the ball club the first year but I can't recall if he played the second. Bill Monbouquette was working again with me and scouting as well for the New York Yankees. Bill always said he liked my mechanics but he did want me to use my legs more. I had an unbelievable fall season that included throwing a no-hitter against Holy Cross. When the game was over, their head coach called me over and offered me a full scholarship. I knew I could play there but didn't think I could handle the everyday grind of the school work. As well as many other schools, the University of New Haven was in pursuits of my talents. To be honest, at the time I had not heard much about the school, but, boy, did I later.

Mo Maloney knew what he had for this coming spring team and he, as well as all of us, was excited. Judy was now potentially in the picture. It started to get better as the year went along. Our season got underway and we got off to a great start. We were beating people pretty good. We had great pitching. Once again the team I was looking forward to facing was North Shore Community College with John Tudor and, of course, Karen. Once again, we would end up playing them toward the end of the regular season. Just before our meeting, I had thrown a no-hitter against Bristol Community College. I think I had given up, maybe two runs the entire year. I had a no-hitter against Johnson & Wales but a windblown popup landed inside the first base line by inches when our first baseman John Greely misjudged it. To this day, he jokes about it with me but I couldn't blame John for anything. He was a great player all around and gave us one hundred percent every time out.

Now was the showdown with North Shore. We knew we were much better than them but we still had to show it on the field. We played them at our park and we jumped out early. We were hitting Tudor pretty well. The first at bat I faced him, I tripled. That put us ahead 1-0. By my next at bat, we were up I think 3-0. I homered in that at bat. My next at bat was a double so by my last at bat I needed a single to hit for the cycle. We were way up by that point and John was still in there. When I walked to the plate, Mo (who was coaching third) called me over and said if you lay down and beat it out for the cycle, I'll give you $10. Well, first pitch was right down the middle and I did push one down third base. I legged it out. By the time I got to third base, Mo said "You owe me $10." I said , "What?" He said he phrased the bet the other way around but I knew he was playing with me. Anyway, we won that one 10-0 and won the second game of the doubleheader to sweep them. We went on to win the state championship again. Tudor ended up having a good career in baseball. He really didn't have the support in his lineup offensively and defensively. I respect him and liked him as a person. A few years later, my sister-in-law Donna was flying for Eastern Air Lines and she met him. She told me he paid me quite a compliment when she mentioned my name. That was nice.

Judy was my prom date and we had a good time but it was time to move on. Although my father really liked Judy, I had to say goodbye. One night during the season, I went out with Karen and we had a bite to eat at a Chinese restaurant. Dad had let me use the car that night. After eating, Karen and I decided to go to Mount Hood in Melrose. It was known to be a parking spot for couples at night. I can't recall why I was low with my blood sugar (I think I gave too much insulin and not enough food) but I was really low. Between the darkness and being low, I hit the boulders on the side of the road and damaged my father's car. I didn't know how I was going to tell him. I couldn't tell him I was at Mount Hood. I told him a car swiped me making a turn and just kept going. Rocco used to call those types of things "white lies." But Dad, as usual, just told me to be more careful next time. Plus, I didn't want him to know I would have low blood sugars while driving the car. He may not let me take it much. He was your "great Dad."

The state championship was next for us again. We played Quinsigamond Community College. They were a junior college power but we got to the championship game at their home park and beat them handily. We were champs again. Soon after that, Harwich of the Cape Cod League wanted me to come down there and try out. I went and threw really hard but at the time I had a job lined up for the summer and I would have to make the move in the next few days so I decided against it.

The Mass. Bay awards dinner was something all the players were looking forward to. Coach Maloney presented me with the Most Valuable Player award. I also was named to the National All-American team as a designated hitter and pitcher. I led the Northeast with 110 strikeouts and 1 run. Coach Maloney had mentioned at the banquet in his speech that I could go on to play for anyone in the country. The University of New Haven was ready to make their offer to me for the next two years. Now I was starting to hear so much about their baseball program and most of all their great coach Frank "Porky" Vieira. His assistant Joe Tonelli came to see me twice during the year and both games I won, 1-0 and 2-0. So he sent Coach "V" down to see me. That game I pitched very well but not like usual. He said our team defense cost me the game with five errors but I wasn't one to make excuses. I always said if the defense is making errors that means the other team is making contact. So, I blamed myself. However, Coach Vieira liked me. He knew I could win at the next level. He offered me a full ride and, because I was so impressed with Coach Tonelli and Coach "V", I took the offer. The one thing he said to me was, "Do you want to be a pro?" I answered "Yes." He said, "Then this is the place to come." He had told me they had Red Sox right fielder Joe Lahoud, Philadelphia Phillies right hander Dave Wallace and Ron Diorio, already in the major leagues at that point.

9.

I Was Now Playing For The Legend, The Greatest Of 'Em All - Vieira

THE SUMMER FOR AUGUSTINE'S ATHLETICS was routinely successful. I wanted to work hard but enjoy myself before leaving home really for the first time. I was dating a girl named Linda who I met in the nightclubs. She was from Revere. Once in a while I would see a local girl, Geri. With Geri and me, it was really just a sexual thing. Linda, I took out quite a bit. The only thing I didn't like about the situation with her was she never got along with her brother. I didn't like that they never even acknowledged each other at home and certainly not at family functions. One night Linda and I were going out. I was supposed to pick her up at a certain time but because I messed up on my insulin intake, I didn't get to her house for at least an hour and a half later. Don't forget, I never tested my blood sugar like I was supposed to. So I never really knew how accurate my insulin dosages were. She was mad. I was seeing three of everything; three green or red lights; couldn't even read the time on my watch. That was a tough night, really tough. Sometimes these lapses with the diabetes could linger for a couple of days.

The next game I pitched, I felt it, but I threw with the best assortment of pitches I had thrown in some time. It was against Winchester. I was throwing "gas" and had maybe the best curveball and slider I can ever remember having. We were winning 1-0 in about the fourth inning. My catcher, Billy Ryan, called for a fastball. Because of my eyesight, I thought he put down three fingers. I threw a changeup and Billy Wolfe, who later became a good friend of mine, jumped on it and hit it out for a home run that tied the score. Ryan came to the mound and asked why I threw a changeup when I had such a great fastball. I told him I read his signal wrong. That's the vision you lose at times with the reaction to the disease. I crossed up Billy two or three other times this game but I got away with them. We won 2-1 and Billy said to the newspapers, "I felt bad for the hitters tonight against Caiazzo. They had no chance."

I struck out twelve in a 6-inning shortened game. Rocco was there and, after the game, gave me some more orange juice he had in the car. During the game, I drank two cans but I don't know why I was still pretty low. After all the games, Mom and Dad would have a big dinner ready on the table for me. Russ came to most games and he would always be invited, and let me tell you, Russ loved my mother and father's Italian cooking and he would feast at the table. Rocco and Russ loved each other. To this day, Russ says, "Your father was the greatest guy I ever came across." He was a regular guy; not one bit of phoniness in him.

As the summer progressed, so did the team. We were cruising along but still had the Hosmer Chiefs close to us. Brother Steve was playing for us again and hitting tremendous home runs. There had just been a big article in the Boston Globe about Steve being at Minnesota and probably going to be the number one flanker for the upcoming season. But after a major knee operation, he chose to bypass his senior year and go right into pro football with the New England Patriots. He was going to be a tight end now that he was 247 pounds. His competition was Russ Francis (Howard Cosell's all-world tight end) and Bob Windsor, the veteran.

The crowds were once again very big no matter where we were playing but especially in those Hosmer Chiefs games. One of the toughest hitters I had trouble with was Bunky Smith from Framingham. He had just been released from the Red Sox. He was just a damn, good hitter. When we were matched up against the Hosmer Chiefs again, I was scheduled to pitch against my old friend Ron Luongo. This was a big game and once again I got a wakeup call from the local paper wanting to know who I thought would win this night and how it revisited the old high school game from a couple of years earlier. I told the writer it was a revenge game. What a crowd! I outpitched Luongo 2-1 in this one. I finished the season a strong seven wins and two losses but more importantly, we won another IC championship. It was fun when we played because everyone you knew was at the game. Even when I wasn't pitching and playing the outfield (right field in particular), the bandstand was situated right behind right field and all the kids I knew hung out there. They'd be talking to me in between innings and sometimes pitches. They'd be drinking and smoking and having a great time. Peter Levine was one kid in particular I knew. He's a big sports fan. Peter was and still is a good guy. He, to this day, still remembers a lot of those games and the players.

The career at the University of New Haven was just beginning. I knew I had to report in tremendous shape and be ready. I had just returned from a St. Louis Cardinal tryout invitation-only camp. After I pitched, the Cardinal brass called me aside and said "you know you are going to the best baseball college there is. Vieira will prepare you for pro ball. If you can play for him, you can play for anyone." People always said you had to have thick skin to play for him. Boy, did I find that out. This guy had eyes in the back of his head. One time we were practicing, and we were running laps and we got to an area where we didn't think coach could see us. It was 95 degrees and I was ready to drop along with a few others. Three other guys and I stopped to walk a few steps and all we heard was "Caiazzo, get it going." But I knew he cared. He was tough as they come. He used to tell me, "When I stop talking to you, that's when you have to worry."

When we were getting into the beginning of our fall games, Coach V told me that Bill Monboquette (Yankee scout) gave him the best recommendation he ever gave anyone. I asked Coach V what Monbouquette said and he stated, "Just give Caiazzo the ball, pull up a chair and sit back and enjoy him pitch." In junior college, when I threw my no-hitter against Holy Cross, I remember Coach Maloney saying to me, "You better throw a good game today because Bill Monbo gave up going to the World Series (Oakland vs. Cincinnati) to come see you pitch."

I was starting to enjoy New Haven. I was living in the New Haven Motor Inn for $25 a week plus they got me a job there, as well. The only thing I was disappointed in was there weren't a lot of girls at the university. Whoever you found, you had to go off campus or go to another school to find them. Although back in the summer I met a friend of Trixie's named Diane. She was a crazy woman but, man, did she like sex. She would come to New Haven to visit for the weekend and we sometimes would never come out of the bedroom. Trixie used to tell me she was tough for a girl. She had 40 DDs and she looked great, but once again, I lost interest eventually.

Just about this time the family got bad news. We lost Noni Matilda, Dad's mother. That was a tough loss. She was wonderful and we all loved her dearly. She was such a great woman. She would give my friends money when I would take them by to visit. Her cooking – Outstanding! That's where my father got his talent from. Her face would light up when she saw all the grandkids. We were going to miss her.

The first game I pitched in the fall I did pretty well but learning to pitch with the pressure Coach V put on you was far more than I could ever expect. Every pitch was important. Something I never dealt with before was getting out of tough situations. I used to think, if I had the bases loaded and no one out but gave up one or two runs, I was doing fine. Not with Coach V. He came up to me once and said, "That's bullshit. Don't you give up anything!" I was learning quickly. There was a game in the fall pitching against Quinnipiac College and I went seven innings, striking out twelve and giving up two hits. After the game, all my teammates gave me a warm "great game Cai." Not Coach V. The next day before practice, he called me over and I thought he's going to say how well I pitched. He said, "I want you to take that curveball and shove it." He wanted me to go with the fastball and slider. He loved that hard, breaking pitch. We were all learning why he was the "Great Vieira." He wouldn't settle for mediocrity. The whole team was in that same mold, though. He would not recruit kids that were good. He wanted them great and wanted professionals or potential pros. The kids were all tough kids having one goal in mind, to be professionals.

While living and working at the Motor Inn, I would see coach quite frequently because he was friendly with Ron Karlins, the manager at the Inn. I would see him for breakfast in the lounge, etc. We hit it off pretty well. I knew he really did like me not only as a pitcher but as a person. But he was "Vieira." He wasn't going to let me get away with anything. He wasn't going to let me know he liked me. I still had to earn everything that eventually was coming to me. We played the University of Maine which had returned from the College World Series the year before. I was pitching and I had struck out the first two batters. Against the third batter, I pumped two fastballs by him and was way up in the count and figured I could do it again. He laced a base hit to left. Vieira came to the mound and said, "If that happens again, you'll never see the mound again." I learned right then and there what I had to do. No mistakes.

10.

Eating Breakfast Every Morning With Hall Of Famer Hoyt Wilhelm

WHEN THE FALL SEASON ENDED, I concentrated a bit more on hitting the books. I made no excuses to anyone. I wasn't an A student but I certainly wasn't a bad one. I just had to really focus on my studies more. What used to happen in class was I would day dream a lot. Somehow, it was always about baseball, thinking of me pitching against a certain team, etc. But I did pretty well with my grades. I also met a barmaid named Wendy who worked at the Motor Inn. She caught my eye as soon as I saw her for the first time. We hit it off pretty easily and she had a friend who waitressed with her named Karen. She would come to the games and loved baseball. She always mentioned how she loved to watch me pitch in my uniform. She was hot. Even Coach V commented on her. When Trixie and Russ and the rest of the guys came out to visit, they were like kids in a candy store around her. Wendy would notice when I became low with my blood sugar. She'd bring me over extra food. She knew I loved the New York cheesecake and never charged me for anything. At the end of her shift one night, she called me and said she was on her way up to my room. She came up and we did our thing. The one thing with Wendy was we didn't go out too often. If we did, it was more like a movie. After all, I was still in school and couldn't afford much.

I started to become friendly with a couple of former major leaguers at the Inn. The New York Yankees AA farm team played in West Haven and the manager was former Chicago White Sox third baseman Pete Ward and his pitching coach was Hoyt Wilhelm, a knuckleballer who pitched for five teams and was the first relief pitcher elected to the Hall of Fame. They were great guys. I would eat breakfast with Pete and Hoyt almost every day. As a kid, I'd watch them on TV a lot. What great players. One day I went down for breakfast and, as usual, picked up the newspaper to read. When I saw the sports page, I read "Wilhelm – A Living Legend." The story covered two full pages. I read it and then, wouldn't you know it, who comes in to sit with me – Hoyt. I said to myself, how am I going to tell him about this in the paper. Of course, he's seen thousands of articles about himself. This, I'm sure, wasn't any different. When he sat down, I said, "Hoyt, there's a nice article in the paper about you." He responded, "OK, I'll see it later." What a nice man. He walked with the right side of his body hanging lower than his left. I think that was due to all the pitching he did. Both Pete and Hoyt became friendly with Coach V. Pete and coach would play racketball together.

Trixie was starting to visit me often and Coach V got the biggest charge out of him. Trixie was a comedian. He had more jokes but he also, at the time, weighed in at nearly 400 pounds. But what a personality. He had what you would call "charm." No matter what he said or did, it was hilarious. I don't know where he got all the jokes from but he kept everybody in stitches. A good friend; one of my best.

After the fall season we had a short break but then we started to work out constantly. While working out inside, we would start to hear stories about Coach V. How great he was as a basketball player in his day. We couldn't believe some of them. As a college player at Quinnipiac, he was considered one of the greatest of all time. He averaged about thirty-two points a game. The biggest story about coach was when he was a senior. He was considered the greatest little man in the game. Coach was only about 5 ft. 8 in. Wilt Chamberlain was the greatest big man in the game. They played against each other in a game in the Catskills and Coach outscored Chamberlain. As coach tells the story, at one point he went underneath Chamberlain's legs and scored. He said Chamberlain wasn't happy about the outcome of the game. During our workouts, coach would at times be shooting jump and hook shots and never missed from way out. I never saw anything like it.

Our southern trip was to Daytona Beach, Florida. We had a tough trip to look forward to playing St. John's University, Fordham, and others. Coach V got us together before the trip and said, "Let's start now to put it in gear. Let's have the same relationship we've always had, you don't talk to me and I don't talk to you, except baseball talk." He meant business

Our spring training trip included all the teams I spoke about and working out with the Montreal Expos. Daytona Beach was their spring training site. Bumping elbows with greats such as Gary Carter (Hall of Fame), Tony Perez (Hall of Fame), Warren Cromartie, Ellis Valentine, Dick Williams (Hall of Fame), boyhood idol Stan Bahnsen, and Rusty Staub was just a dream. Every night we would go to Big Daddy's nightclub and almost all the Expos were there. This was the year Trixie began to really get attached to my teammates and Coach V. He made the trip down south with us. Everyone loved Trixie.

Coach V threw me right into the soup the first game down there. I came out of it nicely. I worked two scoreless innings. The next game he started me and I went five innings only giving up one unearned run. Even though coach was still like a maniac on the sidelines, I was starting to get comfortable around him. I really don't think being comfortable around coach is normal but you know what I mean. When I wasn't getting the strikeouts, I was getting the weak ground balls. My fastball used to sink and tail a lot so I was considered more of a ground ball pitcher than a fly ball pitcher. Pitching twice more down south was about the end of it before coming home. The last game, coach threw me in with the bases loaded and one out, and I got out of the jam and finished the game. We would basically throw two to five innings in Florida to get ready for the regular season. Just before we broke camp, I met a girl down at the strip on the beach. I brought her back to my room for a few hours. My roommate and good friend, Tom Keating, left the room so I could be with her. "Keats" was a fabulous kid, a really great friend, and had a heart of gold. That night with that girl I was about as low as I could be with my blood sugar. I hadn't checked my count but just felt really, really low. After having sex with her, I passed out. Keats, I remember, had to call me to get me up and get him into the room and her out of the room.

Keats was booking a lot in those days. I used to watch him in classes figuring out who owes him what amount of money. I mean, I never saw anything like it. At times, I would ask Tommy, "This guy owe you $15,000?" He would say yes and I would have my mouth open. The number of people on his list and the amount of money was unbelievable. One night, Tommy came by the Motor Inn and asked me to take a ride with him. While in the car, he told me some guy owed him $20,000 and he needed someone to go with him to collect. Of course, I said I'm with him all the way, but to be honest I was a little scared. Didn't know who the person was or what he would do. It was pitch black outside and we pulled up to an open parking lot and there was this big, huge guy sitting in his old Cadillac waiting. Tommy said, "Just stay in the car and I'll be right back. All I could see was Tommy and me getting shot and there goes our lives. I was beginning to get nervous when he didn't come out of the other car for a few minutes. Finally he got out and started to get into our car. I didn't feel safe until we got back onto the parkway heading home. What a scare but Tom said he paid him in full.

11.

"I Love Cai. He's Got Balls"

THE BASEBALL TEAM WAS BACK home now and Coach V gave me and Tom Michalczyk the opening day assignments for the doubleheader. Tom threw a 6-0 game and mine was a 9-1 win. Anyone who knows me knows that confidence was never a question. I was feeling good and had that sense of confidence in my body knowing I was going to succeed at this high level of college baseball. We were beginning to pound teams. We had a relentless lineup. Coach V was dealing with all the hitters and man was he good at it. We had monstrous guys on our team, not small guys. Coach V used to say before we'd even get onto the field we would be up five runs once the opposition saw us walking into the park.

We opened the season something like 12-1. Pat Murphy, our great catcher, would always say to me, "Cai, once I caught you in the fall, I knew you were going to be a big winner for us." One of our coaches who wasn't on the payroll but knew baseball, Bob Cohen, used to call me the Chairman of the Board after Whitey Ford. "Cai, that curve is unhittable," he used to say. Our assistant coach was Joe Tonelli. What a genius on the diamond. Coach V to this day calls him the smartest guy he knows on the field. Joe would take chances at third base as a coach and always come out on top. This guy just studied the game like no one else; knew every rule in the book.

By the midway point in the season, I was feeling great, although at times my arm would act up a bit. When it did, it was painful. I had never thrown so much in all my early baseball career. But I loved the competition and never opted not to go in for relief if coach needed an inning here or there. We were now being considered maybe the best team in New England for sure and also one of the tops in the country. What a pleasure it was to play with these guys and for the Vieiras and Tonellis of the college baseball world. It was all baseball at this point. I eased off the women for a while. My father (Rocco) used to say when he would see a girl, "Boys, that's the prize for success." But he also cautioned us on girls who just wanted to be around a star so they would get some exposure or be in the limelight. I worked too hard to let that happen to me. At this time, I was starting to look at women and say to myself, "Could she be a good future wife or mother" and most of the time the answer was "no." So it became very difficult for me to settle in for any length of time with any girl.

The family would take trips on the weekend to watch the games. By the midpoint of the season, offers from the prestigious Cape Cod League were starting to roll in. A bunch of my teammates had received offers, as well, Tom Michalczyk, Pat Murphy, Don Murelli, Bob Turcio and Dennis Paglialunga. The Harwich Mariners and the Yarmouth Red Sox were in pursuit. However, I turned down both offers because, at the time, the Intercity League was so good. But, to this day, I say it was the biggest mistake I ever made. I saw guys like John Tudor, among others who I knew I was better than and they played there and did pretty well and it paid off for them.

Coach V was really starting to get into it now. As post-season got closer, he became more intense. A guy would get a game-winning blooper for a hit and he would say, "That sucked; swing the bat; that's horseshit." He wouldn't let us settle for being good. He made us great. I've never in my lifetime ever seen a coach as successful as him. One of the few games we were losing, we were down by six runs with one out to go. Coach called the team in and said, "I don't care about the loss if we lose, but we better go down like men, swinging the bats." I never saw anything like it. We kept hitting everything like rockets and pulled out the win. Another time we were down by three runs with one out to go and he said if we don't start swinging the bats, the next day in practice was going to be like the Boston Marathon. Guess what? We won.

As we approached post-season play, keeping up with the control of my diet and medication was important. John Valeri would always ask me if I ate my meals, etc. He was a good kid. He sometimes would spot when I was having a reaction or was feeling off a bit. He was helpful because John lived at the Motor Inn with me. He was my roomie. Plus, I always felt bad that John didn't get to play much at New Haven. He was a very good ball player but he had some unbelievable competition to deal with. Tom Grant (Chicago Cubs) was in right field, Kenny Young (Red Sox) was in center, and Steve Tipa (Chicago White Sox) was in left. When John did get in and got a base hit, Coach V would yell out of the dugout, "Telling us something, Leri?" But he would always be a spot player on that team. Too bad because John was a good kid who worked hard.

One game against Siena College, I pitched a shutout. During the course of the game, I would look in for my sign from Murph and couldn't see it too clearly. This went on the entire game. At points, Murph would come out to the mound and say, "Cai, you crossed me up on that pitch." I wasn't feeling too good that game but pushed myself to get that whitewash. Plus, a lot of scouts were there watching me and a 6 ft. 7 in. first baseman named Gary Holle (Milwaukee Brewers). I handled him pretty well that day. I remember he went zero-for-four against me with two Ks. But, man, after the game the reporters came up to me and I said I don't know how I did this but we got the "W." It was tough. John Stein, a big reporter from the New Haven Register newspaper, was starting to write some great articles about me. One article was about me toughing out a victory and acting like a true professional. At one point in that game, I walked off behind the mound and thought I was going to keel over I was so out of it. But remembered that I was the guy on the hill and wasn't going to let anyone down. This disease wasn't going to get the better of me. Someday maybe but not now. I wasn't going to let that happen. The thing with pitching is you exert yourself so much with each pitch throughout the entire game that you burn off too much energy and can get into that "trance" as I often call it, where you don't know where you are. You're like a drunk. I was starting to forget at times how it feels to feel good for an entire day. It doesn't happen anymore with me. It's a struggle day in and day out, feeling tired all the time. It is tough to just live on a daily basis with no problems concerning diabetes let alone playing a sport at the level of New Haven. But Coach V used to tell people, "I love Cai. He's got balls."

Winning was getting to be like an obsession now. The team didn't want to lose, period. Every time it was my turn in the rotation, I remember telling my roommate Johnny V that I was going to win. One day in the school cafeteria between classes, a student approached me and said, "Cai, I heard you're pitching today. I said, "I am." He said, "Johnny V was telling me New Haven is playing Sacred Heart today and we'll win because every time Cai says he is going to win, he does." You have to have that confidence. You don't want to be too overconfident but I never had too much, just enough. To this day, the Caiazzos get their inner strength from my father, Rocco.

The City Series was taking place at the Yale Bowl. There was Yale, Quinnipiac, Southern Connecticut State and us. It's a yearly thing with the same four teams participating. The Yale Bowl baseball field was beautiful. Ken McKenzie, the former New York Met player, was the head coach at Yale. We breezed through those teams pretty easily but Coach V was still treating each pitch like it was the playoffs. Whether we were up by one run or ten runs, there was no letting up. We won the series but that wasn't our goal. Now we just continued with our regular-season schedule.

When we would play the New York teams, Coach would say to us, "We're not gonna outtalk them but let's outhit, outpitch and outscore them." He referred to them as "those New York bastards." The New York schools had a way of running their mouths. You just had to shut them up.

Coach Vieira's brother Gus, his older brother, who pitched a number of years with the Chicago Cubs organization, was showing me many things on the mound and helping me out tremendously. He was good. Gus was always with a cigarette in his hand smoking constantly. When I would go home for a weekend in the offseason, Gus would stay in my hotel room. At that time he was just coming off a stroke. He was paralyzed on one side of his body and would slur his words. When I would come back from home and get to my hotel room, man, did that room smell like smoke. But I didn't care. He was Gus and Coach V's brother.

As the regular season wound down, we were ranked number one in New England. I was having quite a year. Going into the tournament, I was 10-0. The regionals were held at Springfield College. We got to the final game. I had pitched two days prior and won. We needed this so Coach asked me if I could go with one day rest. Of course, I said "Yes." We played Sacred Heart and they had some power, especially a kid named Joe Rae-tano. I was cruising along pretty good but knew it might just be a matter of time before I lost my strength. Going into the seventh inning, I had a 1-0 lead. Then, all of a sudden, no more zip on the fastball, no more movement, the curveball wasn't biting, and the slider and changeup weren't there for me. We lost and that ended our great season. It was an outstanding season for most of the players, including me, but not for Coach V. He looked forward to the next year the minute we lost. I received some good awards at season's end but not the one we all wanted.

12.

Brother Steve Was Now A New England Patriot

NOW THAT I HAD COMMITTED to the Intercity League instead of the Cape League, I was ready to pick up where I left off. The Augustine's A's team was going to be stacked. We played a couple of pre-season games before we started but we were ready to get it going. Steve Ring had now left the managerial position to Joe DiSarcina. Steve and Joe had played together at UMass. Steve's family business brought him to the Cape. Steve had helped me tremendously and turned out to be a great friend. I had great respect for Steve and owed him a lot. Joe was just a great ball player, as well, and was a great person. As the years went along, I ended up playing with some of the greatest New England shortstops. I don't believe anyone had the ones I had over a career.

On the nights I wasn't pitching, my friends and I would hit the night-clubs. Tony C's was big back then. I met a girl one night there and we went out for the summer. She was from East Boston. She was nice but…you know the same thing happened. I lost interest after a while. Her name was Joanne. She did have a concern about my diabetes. She was making sure I ate well enough and didn't cheat with sweets, stuff like that, but she wasn't what I was after. Never saw her again after the breakup.

My brother Steve was now getting pro football offers. Even though he passed up his senior year at Minnesota, the teams were well aware of his ability. Nobody around these parts had seen this type of talent. Ed Rideout was the only other guy that people were amazed with on the football field.

Steve had tremendous size (6-foot, 3-inch, 246 pounds) and was tough; I mean tough. No one messed with Steve. Besides that, he had about a good a pair of hands as anyone had seen. One University of Minnesota football coach I talked to on the telephone told me how Steve got in a physical encounter with one of his teammates who went on to be an All-Pro in the NFL for a few years. He told me Steve beat him up pretty good in practice one day. Steve was the nicest guy you ever would meet anywhere but…don't cross him. The Dallas Cowboys were sending him letters but the New England Patriots brought the most to the table. Steve was a flanker at Minnesota but NFL people knew with his size, speed and hands, he would make a great tight end. Bob Wolf handled Steve's contract with the Patriots and he was going to report by the end of the summer. The other tight ends were all-world Russ Francis and veteran Bob Windsor. The area was pretty excited about the news on Steve. The only question was whether or not the knee would hold up. Now that he wasn't playing baseball, when he would come down to see me pitch, he was always mobbed with people around him. Being proud of my older brother was nothing new.

Keeping up with my diabetes was a job in itself. Although the family watched over me day to day, I still had to watch myself more carefully. Although I took great care of myself, sometimes I would become stubborn. For instance, when I would be borderline by being normal or low, I would always figure I could make it through the potential "low." You just can't do it. Always thinking I was some kind of "superman" doesn't work. One day I had nothing on my calendar or schedule so I figured I would go to Revere Beach by myself. Unfortunately, I didn't bring any food with me and was just getting sun. Being there for more than six hours, I was so low. I was surprised I could even get up. But I did. Not being able to find my car on the street took more out of me. Finding it was difficult but I did. What a mistake-trying to drive home. I really don't remember much but I do remember ending up in Nahant. Managing to stop at a store I happened to see, I bought some fruit and a bottle of orange juice. Trying to give the cashier money was like a show in itself. He was asking for the correct amount and I kept giving him something short of the amount. He wasn't getting angry but was frustrated. No one was more frustrated than me. I think he realized I had something wrong with me. He opened the juice and told me to drink it. He waited patiently and would not let me go to my car. That was the safe thing to do and he was very nice to do that. Some people could care less. Once I became "normal" again, I got into my car and drove home. When I looked at the time, it must have been two and a half hours that I was driving around in that physical state. That could have been a very dangerous situation.

The A's season started off the way everyone expected – winning. The Hosmer Chiefs were winning, as well. So when it came time to play them head on, it became fun. The league started an all-star team, as well, to play the famous Boston Park League. But that was a few weeks away. There were some good pitchers in our league so I knew I had to stay on my game. Our team was a big thing in town. No matter where you'd go, people would be stopping us and asking us about the games and talking baseball. When it was time to play the Chiefs, everyone was surprised to hear that I wasn't getting the start. Joe had decided to pitch Rich Rappoli. Everyone in the league, let alone our team, knew I was the ace of the staff so no one was more surprised than me. Joe and Rich were friends from way back to their teenage years. Some people questioned whether it was because of that. As always, though, I wanted the ball. The Chiefs were going with their ace, Jeff Williamson, so why shouldn't I get the ball? The players all knew I was as much a team player as you would want but also knew that decision wasn't going to go over well with me. Thinking about it over and over again, I said I wasn't going to say much until I saw the result. Rappoli got ripped and only lasted a short time. When he came out he ended up sitting next to me on the bench and he never stopped complaining about his arm hurting and how sore it was. I mean it was so sore, according to him, I even said he should get it looked at by someone. The one thing I never did was "make excuses." It seemed to a few of our players that he was making excuses for his ineffectiveness. After the loss to the Chiefs, the next game I approached Joe before the game. I was angry but I was professional. I told him he shouldn't have made the pitching decision he did. Joe O'Donnell, the Chiefs player-coach, had been pursuing me to play for them but now I was thinking maybe I should switch. It was still early in the season and if I chose to, I could make the change. When Joe didn't give me the answer I was expecting, I told him I either play with the A's and we win it or go to the Chiefs and they win it. I was showing my cockiness but that was me. I started to walk away and Joe kind of followed me and said it wouldn't happen again and he knew I was the ace and didn't want me to leave. I got all the big game starts after that.

Bob Corcoran was our other big game pitcher. I loved Bob and whenever he got the call I never minded. Shortly after the Chiefs game, Rappoli came back to pitch maybe only two games later and he went the distance to win. It was like his arm never bothered him. I pitched all my life and knew if someone's arm bothered them that much, you couldn't pitch for some time let alone a couple of days later. That was something a lot of our players were not comfortable with. I realized I had business to take care of and wasn't going to let that incident bother me. My head was screwed on right and I kept winning my every start.

When the all-stars were selected, a several members of the A's were selected. The Park League had some great players I had read about for years. Don January, who later on in years I became good friends with, was one. He was a former farm hand of the Red Sox. Paul Winnick, a great left-hander for years and a farm hand of the Washington Senators, was another. The game was played at Trum Field in Somerville. We had some great players of our own, guys such as Joe DiSarcina, Billy Ryan, Bob DeFelice, Jack Repetto, Joe O'Donnell, Ed Rideout, Charlie Meeker, Dave Polcari, Bob Corcoran, Mark Santini and Jeff Williamson, among many others. We won that game on a one-sided affair. I pitched two scoreless innings. What I remember most was facing Don January and striking him out on a slider down and away. My catcher was Bob DeFelice, a former Red Sox farm hand himself who knew January very well. He told me he was a great fast-ball hitter so when I got ahead of January I went with the hard breaking ball.

Dad's business was starting to get worse. He and Mom had sold the house on Rockland Avenue and bought a two-family on Maple Street. His health was still shaky. It wasn't good to have his health like that at the same time his business was on shaky ground, as well. Mom was now working at Gillette Company in South Boston now that Kennedy's Clothing had gone out of business. She was working as an inspector in the razor blade section. She worked hard, on top of being a great Mom.

Dad did have another setback with his heart. He was back in Mass. General Hospital again with another heart attack. This one, however, wasn't as bad as the first one. He was in the hospital for at least a week. Each time I'd go to visit him I'd have tears in my eyes and would give him a big hug and kiss. My family didn't want to see him suffer. He was as tough as they come, though, and battled through this one, as well.

13.

I Don't Take Advice From Anyone Who Hasn't Done It

A FRIEND I WENT TO school with was starting to go to some of the clubs and we got together a number of times with some of our friends. Through him I met a girl, Joyce, who I started to date. She was very pretty and had an outstanding body. She did some modeling. At the time I started to see her, she was a manager at a health club. We were seeing each other maybe twice a week. After a couple of weeks, we went out to get a bite to eat. Afterward, she asked me if I wanted to see the health club she worked at. The place was closed but she had a key. It was very late at night. She opened the doors and once we got one foot inside, the music went on really loud. She ran to turn it off. It probably was on a timer. As she showed me around, she started to get a bit affectionate. Things developed and next thing you know we were on one of the mats that were on the floor. I knew sooner or later something would develop with us. Joyce was a nice girl. We got along pretty well. She was into the athletes. She had a sister who was every bit as attractive as Joyce. Joyce looked tremendous in her jeans and her sister might have looked even better in hers. I was starting to sleep around a little too much but I was at that age where anything that looked good was a challenge. But I was always careful when I slept with someone; made sure I had protection. I had the fear, also, of not pleasing someone because of the diabetes problem. It was a known fact that diabetics had trouble either getting it up or keeping it up. My doctor would always ask me each time I went to see him. Most girls, I didn't even tell them. I was more embarrassed than anything, So, if I had a problem in bed, it made it more embarrassing

There was a guy who used to always come to our summer games and always showed a complete interest in me, calling me aside to see how I felt and what my thought process was during the game. He was a hell of a guy; real genuine. I appreciated it. But I was a guy who never liked to take advice from just anyone. I only took it from guys who had a good background; who had some history to them. When I asked who he was, Joe DiSarcina said his name was Billy Stathouse from Somerville who was a pitcher with the Minnesota Twins organization. We hit it off great, and I let him know how much I appreciated what he was doing for me and that I was going to respond to his helpfulness. A lot of people lend their advice but if they don't have the history to them, then I don't want it sent to me. There are a lot of people out there who think their word to someone means something but it doesn't mean anything if it doesn't come from some type of creditable source. My thinking has been, if you haven't done it then I don't want you to share with me. My parents always taught me to watch who you take advice from. To this day, I always remember that. There are too many people out there with no credibility.

Steve was getting ready to leave for Patriots training camp soon. At the same time, the A's were ready for another playoff run. We had that power-house team. Our infield, anchored by Joe D at short, was outstanding, as was our pitching and outfield. Our team just never thought the Chiefs, nor anyone else, was better than us, and they weren't. When it came time for the playoffs, we showed our respect to the other teams but we knew we shouldn't lose. If Hosmer threw the top three pitchers and were on top of their game, they could dominate teams. Bobby Corcoran and myself didn't fear anyone and did welcome whoever's ace was pitching against one of us. We both had that same makeup. Bobby was the nicest guy you could meet. He was classy, smart naturally (he was a Yale guy), funny and a gamer. He was also a dignified-looking man. When he was between those lines, he was serious. He was like a different person when pitching as opposed to being on the bench talking it up to whomever was pitching that day. I respected him tremendously; my type of player and person.

When the A's were going through the semi-finals pretty easily, we knew we were going to eventually get matched up in the finals again with the Chiefs. They had a scary lineup with guys such as Dave Polcari, Eddie Rideout, Bob DeFelice and Joe O'Donnell. But our lineup was fierce. We went seven games in the championship series with Freddy Campatelli having a great series and Joe DiSarcina simply being Joe, no one better at the shortstop position. The seventh game was a great one.

Steve had just been released from the Patriots after a pretty good showing but knew his time might be short with his bad knee injury recurring.

When I went to see him at training camp, he showed exceptional hands but his mobility wasn't what it was in the past.

Now it was "get ready" for my big year at New Haven. We had everyone returning for my final year. Our expectations were high, as were everyone's opinions on how we were going to do once the bell rang. Fall baseball was very successful and I ended up winning three or four games in about a twelve- or thirteen-game schedule. The staff of myself, Tom Michalzyck (Chalz), Tony Notorino and Jerry Perry was ready to go. From the previous year, we kind of figured Tommy and I were going to get the bulk of the work again. We were ready. Coach V and Coach Tonelli worked us hard in the fall. I was feeling pretty strong and knew I had to keep a close watch on my sugar. I had to follow my diet as closely as possible and not abuse my body. Wendy was back at the hotel again and that to me was both good and bad. I just knew I had to keep control of myself and know when to say "go" or "no."

One of my very close friends on the team Tommy Keating (Keats) and I had received word that we were named co-captains for the 1977 team. Tommy was a tough, hard-nosed infielder who, back in high school, was a three-sport standout playing basketball and also football as an all-state linebacker. Being named a co-captain on this particular squad made me feel exceptionally proud due to the members we had. What a team we were expecting to have and to be one of the two main leaders made me feel great. Coach V knew Tommy and me from the previous year so he only pitched us sparingly in the fall. The more of Coach V I saw, the more I couldn't believe how great he really was. I saw more and more how he was so successful over the years. Nobody was in his class as a coach. I mean nobody! He was winning award after award. One night he invited me to his house for dinner with his family in Woodbridge, a town I had never seen around the parts of Boston I grew up in. His house was something else. I could not believe the trophy cases in his house. Just amazing. I always thought my trophies were something to look at but they were nothing next to Coach's. I remember seeing the one trophy I had heard about since the day I stepped foot on the New Haven campus. It was the largest trophy I had ever seen. It went from the floor to the ceiling. So many of the trophies were for basketball as well as baseball. His wife Barbara and his daughters were very cordial to me and treated me like a son or brother. That was very nice to experience.

After the fall season, I was back working a little more at the New Haven Motor Inn again. Seeing Wendy on and off was a regular thing. One night a girl came into the lounge at the Inn with a girlfriend of hers. I got talking to them but I kind of liked one of them. At the same time I was thinking of Keats. So I asked her to go out some night and set Keats up with her friend. We had the weirdest night out with them. As the night went along, I found them both to be a bit strange. Tom Keats agreed. I remember we went to see the movie "Rocky." Keats really got into it; so much so that he didn't pay much attention to the girl he was with. I ended up taking the girl out one more time but Keats never went out again with his girl. Keats and I joked about that night for a long time after that. The girl I was with lived in a very bad neighborhood and, believe me, I didn't want to go back there even though she was a good-looking girl. A few weeks after I took her out for the second time, she came back to the lounge but I talked just a bit to her. She asked me why I hadn't called her back but I made up some excuse to her and that was the end of that relationship.

Russ, Trixie and a bunch of the guys were coming down to visit from Malden quite frequently. We would go to the Yale Bowl to see the New York Giants play because they were using the Bowl as their home field while Yankee Stadium was being refurbished. Other times we would go to New York to visit. One weekend Carl, my old high school catcher, came to visit. What a nightmare! As you know, I worked at the hotel so I had one of the fulltime workers, Billy, set up a function room for us to go back to at night to watch football. I remember Russ went out to pick up a couple of pizzas and Carl took the trip with him. He got Russ so distracted while driving that Russ slammed the brakes on. The pizzas were on the back seat. When the car came to a screeching halt, the pizzas went flying and were everywhere in the car. Russ was tearing mad at Carl. We eventually got something else to eat. When they got back to the Inn, Carl ended up getting into an argument with Billy and I had to separate them. Really stupid. But that was what I had to face every time Carl was around. Constant problems. I always said he would start a fight with someone lying in a casket. He was getting to be such a nuisance, I was losing patience more each time I saw him.

Back in Malden, the Caiazzo household seemed fine. Everyone was getting prepared for our upcoming baseball season. Steve was now starting to hear from the Canadian Football League; the Toronto Argonauts, in particular. Joan was starting to think about Jones College in Florida. She did decide to go but once she got there, she didn't like it at all. She only stayed a few weeks and decided to leave. She really didn't like the area nor the people she was living with. I thought school would be great for her and would really have helped her along the way to prepare for life in general. Joan was still our little sister and we wanted to look out for her. Being the sister and not always getting the attention her big brothers got because of being in the sports page every night made it difficult for her but she was proud of Steve and me.

Angeline and Rocco were making their periodic weekend visits to New Haven with the usual car load of food, mostly homemade pasta, lasagna and meatballs and sausage. Boy, did I miss that! When they came to the New Haven Motor Inn, my roommate Johnny Valeri's eyes would light up because he knew he was going to eat well for the next week or so with Italian food. I loved it when they came to visit. I'd bring them to a great pizza parlor called Ernie's Pizza not far from the hotel. We'd sit for a couple of hours and relax and enjoy the talk of how family was doing. The owners were very nice people and told Mom and Dad how they enjoyed my visits there and they commented how handsome and beautiful Ann and Rocco were. That always made me feel special but especially when they said what wonderful people they were. I knew that, of course, but that always makes you feel even more special to have parents like that. I was as proud of them as they were of their parents. Mom would always talk about how beautiful her mother (Grandma Theresa) was and talk about how the fight game nearly killed her father (Grandpa Joe). He was a professional boxer who, my mother always said, got punch drunk from so many hits to the head. I could barely remember him because he died so young. And Dad would always speak so much about his father (Noni Nick) and mother (Noni Matilda). I remember them more so because they lived much longer lives than Mom's parents.

The older I get, the more I miss those days. They will never come back. I always say that life is basically just memories; and those are memories I'll never forget.

Diane from Winthrop was starting to visit quite a bit again and, once again, it wasn't what I was looking for long-term; just sexual. She was a nice girl, though. I enjoyed her company.

Johnny Valeri and I were in the Motor Inn lounge one night and I got talking to a cute black girl who was by herself. She asked if I knew anyone who wanted to pimp her off. I was shocked. I wasn't interested but Johnny was so I said I would have to try her in bed in order to judge her. She accepted. Don't forget, we were young and did some crazy things. Johnny snuck into the room and I didn't know it but while I was having sex with her, he was hiding in the bathroom. He later told me (after she left) that he watched everything through the mirror on the wall. The next day the girl came back to the lounge and I arranged for her and John to use the room. John kind of liked her but from what I remember, that was as far as that went. He was a good kid.

Trixie was thinking of making the trip to Daytona Beach with the team for spring training. Of course, not just anyone could do that but Coach V took a liking to him and gave the OK for Trixie to come down to Florida with the team. Coach just got a real charge out of him. I'll never forget that before Trixie came with us, his mother gave him about forty miniature bottles of different spirits to take down with him. She worked in a package store so she packed them away for him to take on the flight. Coach V loved his before-, during- and after-meal cordials so that was perfect for him. Trixie would have them on top of the dresser in our hotel room and Coach went through them all in a few days but he never got drunk. During the Florida trip, we were out at the pool in between double sessions and we saw a blind man walking while searching with his cane trying to find his room. Trixie noticed him and asked if he needed some help. The man said yes so Trixie brought him to his room and opened the door for him. Just before he got to the room, the blind man slipped on dog manure and Trixie was helping him take off his shoe. When he came back to us at the pool, Coach Tonelli said, "What happened with that guy?" Trixie told us he stepped in dog shit. Coach started laughing and said, "A fine Samaritan you are. You lead a blind man into dog shit." Coach Tonelli was quite a guy with a great disposition. He, as well, loved Trixie.

Just weeks before leaving for Daytona Beach, Coach V would have scouts, etc., come to the gym during our indoor workouts to teach us additional fundamentals and talk baseball to the team. Guys such as Tom Giordano (who became head of baseball operations for the Baltimore Orioles) would come in. He was so knowledgeable. They would watch our workouts and get a good look at us, as well. These scouts had great respect for our program, and even more so for Coach V.

Before we took our spring training trip to Daytona Beach, I came home one last time to gather up some things because I knew I wasn't coming home again until school and the baseball season came to an end. I went to the Joslin Clinic in Boston to get checked out and make sure everything was fine with the diabetes. One of the important people came up to me and asked if I would speak to a group of diabetics who were very young in age. She wanted me to speak about playing sports at such a high level and being able to overcome any talk on the streets or wherever about not being able to play organized sports. It was to encourage them but I just felt that where I was just a college player at that time, I shouldn't be speaking in a forum any time. So I told her I appreciated the offer but I declined. I guess I should have done it, but I didn't.

14.

Our New Haven Chargers Powerhouse Team Was At It Again

SPRING TRAINING BACK IN FLORIDA was what I was looking forward to. However, just before we left, I pitched in a scrimmage game and felt a twinge in my arm. I started to get worried. One thing I didn't need at this time was arm trouble, especially considering the time of year. I approached Coach V on the situation. What he suggested to do was go out and see the Yale doctor right down the street from us at New Haven. He said he was supposed to be the best in the country. He called me personally and set up the appointment to see him. The next day I was in his office. What he told me was that I had tendonitis in my shoulder. He quickly decided to give me a cortisone shot knowing I had to be in Florida in just a couple of days. Man, when I saw that syringe it made my insulin syringe look like a threading needle. That's how big it was. It seemed that he had the syringe in my arm for a long period of time, pulling it out and redirecting in different locations while injecting the cortisone in me. When he finished, I felt like I was going to pass out. He sent me into a room to lay down for a while. When I came out of the room, I asked him how much cortisone he used. All he said was, "Let's just say I gave you the largest dosage I've ever given anyone." I had no problems with the arm after that all season.

Trixie came to meet me the day before we were leaving for down south. The morning we got to the school to catch the bus to head to JFK Airport something amazing happened. We were all waiting for Tommy Keating (co-captain) to arrive but he was extremely late. Coach V wasn't too happy.

When he arrived, we found out someone blew the whistle on him for his book-ing. Tom had been doing it for some time. I used to see him taking people's debts in a notebook in classes. I couldn't believe the amounts. This particular day, Tom asked some guy who owed him some heavy money to meet him at a restaurant to pay him. Well, I guess what happened was that the guy called the police and reported him and told them where he was going to be and they nabbed Tom. Somehow they let him go but they took his vehicle and all the paperwork he had. So that was something Tommy was going to have to face soon down the road. For the team, the most important thing was that he was still coming to Florida. I felt bad but I loved Tommy.

When we got to Florida, it was all business. Baseball was everyone's main objective. We continued to train just as we did the year before with the Montreal Expos. They had great teams those years with Dick Williams managing, Andre Dawson, Warren Cromartie, Gary Carter, Larry Parrish, Rusty Staub, Ellis Valentine, Billy Gullickson and Doc Edwards.

We were staying in the same hotel with them and that was quite a thrill for young kids. Every night after dinner we would go to Big Daddy's night-club just next door to our hotel and we were with them every night. One day Coach V just wanted me to get my arm checked with trainer Renee and that day Billy Gullickson was sitting next to me on the trainer's table. What a nice guy he was.

Tommy McDonald, Red Sox scout, one night called my room to find out where Coach V was. It must have been around 1 a.m. but I certainly wasn't going to wake up Coach for anyone. Mr. McDonald was a really nice guy. I guess he did get in touch with Coach that evening or morning and they were putting those drinks down from what I heard. Tommy scouted me in high school and junior college and was looking at a bunch of our guys. We had major talent.

The games in Daytona were going to begin so I knew I had to be on top of my game. We had team curfew around 11 p.m. or midnight, depending. The diabetes can really drain a person and when you overdo it to any extent, you're time is limited. I wanted to produce the numbers I always loved – No Runs, No Hits, Just wins! When you're pitching, especially, I had to really watch my intake of the amount of insulin needed. You burn off so much energy that you can get so low with your blood sugar that you need to drink juice or eat sugar during each inning. Dad was the best for bringing that when I was growing up. He always had those cans of orange juice ready.

We were going to play St. John's University and Fordham, as well as some schools from the Midwest during the southern trip. It seemed once you got into that Florida air that sleep wasn't needed as much as when you're around the northern part of the East Coast. I could get four hours sleep but yet feel strong as ever.

Coach V made some moves but nothing drastic from the previous year since most everyone was back. One major change was moving Don Murelli from first base to his natural position at shortstop. He was something to watch. He had that long athletic body with a cannon for an arm. You never, ever would see Don not hustle. We called him "Relli." He would hit a one-hopper back to the pitcher and run down the first base line like Pete Rose. He was a complete ball player. Relli was one of my closest friends on the team. We just "jelled." Coach V was such a great hitting instructor he continuously worked with Don to make him a great hitter. The other change was to move Tom Riley from shortstop to first base. Tom was a little erratic with his glove and arm, although he had one of the best arms I ever saw.

Pat Murphy, our great catcher, was a mainstay, as was Dennis Paglialunga at third and Tommy Keating at second. The outfield was outstanding. All three went on to pro ball. Steve Tipa was in left, Kenny Young in center and Tom Grant in right. Tipa signed with the Chicago White Sox, Kenny Young signed with the Red Sox and Tom Grant with the Chicago Cubs. Coach Tonelli and Coach V used to say Kenny outruns the baseball. Grant had one of the strongest arms I've ever seen. He got his first major league hit off Hall of Famer Tom Seaver years later.

We had an excellent trip and maybe lost one game but played well enough to realize we were a powerhouse again. But this year even better than last.

The previous year I finished at eleven wins and only one loss; the one loss coming at the expense of pitching on one day's rest. When I got my first start of the 1977 season, I lost 1-0 The run scored on a half swing blooper after an error and a stolen base. So I started out 0-1 which I wasn't too happy about. That day the Central Connecticut pitcher threw a great game, kept us off balance and scattered about eight hits. As I stated earlier "I HATED TO LOSE." It just wasn't in my makeup, nor did I get into any routine for that stuff. I prided myself on WINNING. Many times I would think about other players and wondered how they could go about pitching at a 50 percent winning percentage, even 75 percent for that matter. If that was me, I would have been long gone, either quitting the game or committing suicide.

The team went on a pretty good run at this point. We were crushing teams. Coach V used to say teams would look at us and be automatically down 5-0. Most teams were intimidated by us. We basically were all big in size, as well. One game we played Fairfield University and one of their players said they had just played Boston College the day before and he thought they were great but he said we would destroy them. That's how good we were.

My earned run average was at about 1.00 at this point and I had now reeled off about six wins in a row. I was leading the New England pitchers in record and ERA. My teammate Tom Michalczyk also was among the leaders in New England. Tom was great. He really knew how to pitch. He was a great teammate and friend as well, always pulling for everyone and giving positive feedback. "Chalz" played in the Cape League for two years with Dennis Pags, Pat Murphy, Kenny Young and Tom Grant.

One game in particular I was looking forward to was the Sienna game. They had a huge first baseman, about 6 ft. 7 in., named Gary Holle. He was an eventual big leaguer with the Milwaukee Brewers. I was hearing some amazing stories about him along with him being looked at by almost every big league team. That game was soon approaching and I wanted the ball for one of the games of the doubleheader. It didn't take a genius to figure out there was going to be a ton of scouts at the game. Well, the day was finally here and I got the ball in game one. Not only myself but the entire club was juiced up for these two games. The ballpark of ours was packed with both fans and scouts; I saw about fifteen at this game. From experience, I knew these scouts wanted to see strikeouts and velocity. Holle batted third so I faced him in the first inning. I handled him pretty well. I sawed off his bat with a little popup to first base. The next two times I struck him out. On the last at bat I remember having him 0-2 before getting the count even trying to get him to swing at something out of the strike zone. On the 2-2 pitch, I threw him a hard slider down and away and he topped a weak ground ball back to me and that was his day; mine was satisfying. We won pretty good, something like 6-0. They only had a couple of hits and I had about eleven strikeouts.

Another big game was against Eastern Connecticut State. Those in-state rivalries are great. I had pitched the day before and in the Eastern game I was called on in the ninth inning to put out a big threat. The situation was the bases filled and one out. I got a strikeout and got the next batter to bounce out to Murelli at first. That was a big jam to squeeze out of. We went in to the twelfth inning when Tommy Grant hit a big three-run homer to tie the game then Mike Medeiros (not one of our regulars) pinch hit and knocked in the winning run with a single to center field. Coach was ecstatic. When he comes charging out of the dugout with his fist clinched, you know he's fired up.

The sports writers were covering us pretty steadily now that we were winning consistently and getting close to playoff time. They would even be at our practices. I had about nine wins by now and the New Haven Register newspaper sports writers were calling me quite frequently for stories.

We had only one or two games left before we were going to the regional tournament in Syracuse, N.Y. We were top-seeded going into the tourney. The other teams were LeMoyne College, C.W. Post and one other team. We opened up with C.W. Post. They were always tough. Coach V used to tell us we'd better outplay them because "no one can outtalk these New York bastards." We got a kick out of some of his statements. Coach put an article in the paper saying he was opening up the tournament with Caiazzo because he's been throwing the ball best right now. I went the full nine innings and won 4-1. I started out a bit shaky but settled down. Going nine innings is what we were supposed to do. Today's pitchers can't even go four; the game has changed so much. The tournament was extremely tough. We got through the tourney now to face LeMoyne in the big game. The winner would go to the College World Series in Springfield, Illinois. One of the New York Yankees, Daryl Jones, who I became very friendly with when we were both at the New Haven Motor Inn, was going to watch me pitch since Coach V called on me to pitch this huge game. Also in attendance was going to be the Syracuse pitching coach Hoyt Wilhelm and manager Pete Ward, both of whom were promoted by the Yankees to AAA.

Everyone was on good behavior the night before of course knowing the importance of this game. We were ready. When I was coming out of my room, at the Ramada Inn hotel where we stayed, to catch our bus to the park, I was met by Coach Vieira at the elevator. As the elevator was approaching our floor, Coach turned to me and said, "Cai, I just want you to know both the university and especially myself appreciate all you have done for us here, no matter what happens today." I thought, "He must be crazy or something. I'm winning today and our Chargers baseball team is going to the College World Series." As we were getting off the elevator at the lobby, I turned to him and said, "Don't worry, Coach, we're winning today."

We all got to the ballpark (McArthur Stadium) early for pre-game infield and batting practice, etc. We were all pretty raring to go. Pat Murphy, our great catcher, came to me as we were walking out to the bullpen. He said, "Super Chief, I know you'll throw a masterpiece." "Super Chief" was a nickname I got from one of the scouts and part-time coaches for us named Bob Cohen. As I was warming up in the bullpen, I could feel the heat. It was projected to be in the upper 90s so it was going to be a tough

one, not only with the weather but also with LeMoyne. But once again, neither the team nor I was taking a back seat to anyone. We came out swinging the bats and scoring a couple of early runs. Each inning was brutal with
the heat. Bob Deobel, our trainer, was taking good care of me between
innings with ice and cold towels. I got into the last of the ninth and we were
up 6-0. I struck out the first batter. I knew we had this game but I started to
tire a little and walked a hitter who then advanced to second on a wild pitch.
There was a ground ball to shortstop and Don Murelli, who was as slick a
fielder as you'd see anywhere, booted it allowing LeMoyne's only run to
score. When he boots a ball you should take a picture of it because you may
not see it happen again. He was something, although we joked about it later.
I finished it with a ground ball to Paggy at third and we did it.

Coach V always said, "Act like it is supposed to happen." We did but we
also celebrated. As a matter of fact, in the clubhouse we received two cases
of champagne from Pete Ward and Hoyt Wilhelm.

The next day's newspaper in New Haven read "Caiazzo is king." It was
written by the great sports writer Jon Stein. He talked about how Coach V
was nervous before the game and Dave Caiazzo wasn't. Then how I gave
my insulin shots each day to control my diabetes. It was a great article.

15.

Winning The Opening Game Of The College World Series In Caiazzo Fashion

UP TO THAT POINT IN my life, there was nothing that compared with winning that game against LeMoyne because that meant we were going to the College World Series. When we got back to New Haven from Syracuse, everyone was excited for us. Newspaper and sports talk shows were all covering our progress. We worked out at our ball park for a few days before we boarded the bus and plane for Springfield, Illinois. Two days before we left, Coach V announced I was getting the opening game assignment against Shippensburg State from Pennsylvania. My entire family and friends were all excited when they got the news. The local paper (the Malden News) contacted me for an interview. The one thing that I said was that this was nearing the end of my college career but I wasn't going to end early or without flair. That I made sure of.

When we arrived in Springfield, there wasn't much to do other than play baseball. I think that's what the NCAA officials are thinking, as well, when they name a city for the World Series. We just knew it was the Land of Lincoln. From our hotel, we weren't too far away from his childhood home. The very first night we all went to where the other teams were going – a bar, of course. When we were there relaxing, some very attractive women were arriving, as well. There were about fifteen of us at this long table. After an hour or so, two beautiful women came in, one much prettier than the other. One of our guys said, "Look at those two." When we all looked over, they were sitting a couple of tables from us. As a little time went by, our big designated hitter Bobby Turcio, who Lemoyne Coach Rockwell called the best hitter he'd seen at the college level, started to talk to them and invited them over to our table. They came over. We all got talking. After a couple of hours things were developing. Bobby especially liked the really good-looking girl named Melinda. He was doing his best to make some headway with her but I think she was showing to most of us she had an interest in me. As we began to leave the bar, I asked her if she wanted to go to our first game of the World Series. This was going to be New Haven against Shippensburg State. I told her I was going to be pitching that day. She gave me her telephone number and said she loved baseball and would love to go.

The next day was a practice day before the first game so we got out of practice fairly early. When we got back to the hotel, I called Melinda and she invited me to go to a restaurant with her and wanted to show me around the town. She picked me up at the hotel and we went to a Pizza Hut. She was very nice and worked for Teachers Insurance Company in Springfield. I had her bring me back early because the biggest game of my life was the next day.

When I got back to my room, the telephone was blinking showing I had a message. I went to the front desk and there was a telegram sent by Joe O'Donnell, coach of the Hosmer Chiefs, wishing me luck in the series, Joe always wanted me to pitch for him. Joe was one of the most respected businessmen in the country. That was one of the nicest gestures I'd ever seen. What a true gentleman. Years later, Joe was best friends with President George Bush and was seen constantly with him.

The World Series was first class all the way. Our game was the opener for the Series. It began at noon and we were shuttled to the ball park (Lamphier Park). From what we had heard, the park had just been remodeled. It originally was opened in 1928 and seated 5,000 people. It was the home park of the St. Louis Cardinals farm club, but I didn't care what park it was. I was determined to win at anyone's cost, and I knew that was Shippensburg State. I hated to lose. That wasn't going to happen. I would have loved for Mom, Dad, Steve and Joan to be out there to experience the Series but I also knew times were a little tough back then and it wasn't affordable. If I could, I would have paid for them but I was only a college student. The next best thing was for me to win the game and then call home with the good news. But I had a lot of work to do on the mound before all of the other stuff could happen.

Melinda came to the game. I didn't know where she was sitting but I was too focused on the game to even look for her. Once the game started, it was typical New Haven Charger baseball. Coach V was in on every pitch and you could hear his every comment. Nothing was different. Sometimes I would sit there and say, "I wish other kids could experience the joy of being where I am but I was the lucky one. I earned it." Even though I wasn't a pro as yet, I was getting paid to play a game I loved and doing something most people dreamed of. My brother Steve and the family had just called me before I left the hotel to wish me luck. Steve knew how much I wanted this one. We always competed against each other like we were enemies but we were still brothers first. Once the games ended we were back to being brothers and hanging out.

When we were growing up, Steve used to tell me things that made a lot of sense. Although we were a lot alike in many ways, we were older brother and younger brother. Steve was always looking to protect me if there were any problems. But I wasn't a troublemaker so that really did not need to be addressed. He knew, as our entire Caiazzo family knew, that blood is thicker than water. We always spoke about it and Steve would say to me if we had a disagreement that he didn't really like a lot of people he may have appeared to like. He said, "Do you really think I like these people?" Some, yes, but not all of them. We always joked about some people that thought we liked them but really didn't.

Once that National Anthem was playing and we were out on the first base line, the adrenaline was starting to flow. Getting ahead of the hitters was the key. I got the second pitch strike after the first pitch I threw was called a ball. I thought it was right there but the umpire didn't. After the first pitch, I walked in toward home plate and asked for a new ball. The ump said "you only threw one pitch." I said, without anyone noticing or showing him up, that I was going to be there all day long. He gave me everything for the rest of the game.

We got some runs but only two were needed as we won 6-1. The lone run was scored late in the game. When we got to the ninth inning, I said to myself, "Follow what Coach V always preached to us. Act like it's supposed to happen." I finished up strong retiring the side in order with a strikeout mixed in. After the final out, I walked off shaking everyone's hand and that was "it." The reporters had Coach V and I for a post-game interview in the dugout. When they asked Coach about me, he said, "I just call him a pro. Goes about his work on the mound in a professional manner and never gets rattled." The reporter asked me about being related to Joe Pepitone. They found out all the inside information beforehand.

Next we were going to play Eckert College from Florida. They were a powerhouse with future major leaguers Joe Lefebvre and Steve Balboni (nicknamed "The Condominium"). Tom "Chalz" pitched the game and got hit pretty good. They had tremendous power in that lineup. Balboni hit two home runs and Lefebvre had a tremendous game (he was the World Series MVP that year). What an arm he had, as well. Stan Saleski, who later pitched in the Yankee chain, beat us. He was pretty good. We got beat by about eight runs.

We were down after that defeat but had to play in the late morning the next day against Delta State of Mississippi. They were coached by former Red Sox Hall of Famer Dave "Boo" Ferris. Tony Notarino was scheduled to pitch for us. Coach told me I'd be going the next game against eventual champion Cal Riverside if we got to that game. This game moved along pretty well and it was a one-run game and we were losing something like 3-2. I was hanging in the bullpen just in case when the bullpen phone rang. Coach V asked me if maybe I could face two batters, at the most, if necessary. I said yes. He brought me in with the bases loaded and one out with the score now 4-2. I was angry we were losing and close to being eliminated. I looked at the hitter and he was grinning at the third base coach as he was looking down for a sign. I took a step forward and kind of pointed in his direction to get back in the box. I didn't like the smiling part. He got in and I struck him out on three pitches. Now the next batter got in the box and I threw him a slider which he swung at and missed, a fast ball for strike, and then a slider down and away that he missed, and I got out of the jam. But we didn't score in the ninth and lost. We were going home.

Just before the game started, we were hanging in the dugout and one of our guys said "look at that who just said down behind home plate in the red blouse." We all looked and Bobby Turcio said, "She's here to see me." But Tommy Keating interrupted and said, "I have news for you, she's here to see Cai." It was Melinda. Once you lose, the NCAA rushes you right out of town. Coach told us we had a flight in three hours and had to be packed and ready to go home. When we got outside the stadium, I was the last guy to board our van with our private driver. Someone asked me if I got Melinda's telephone number and I said, "No." They said "are you crazy?" I told the driver to stop the van and I would meet everyone back at the hotel. I ran out and went up to where Melinda was sitting in the park and exchanged numbers. She drove me back and it was a relief that I did that. Not too long after the season, Melinda came to Boston for a week and we had a great time. All my friends and family thought she was such a nice girl with the looks to match. I stayed in touch with her for a short period of time after that but up until the time I signed professionally, we lost contact for about eight or nine years until we spoke again.

Once we got back home, the awards for the season were being distributed. I was happy and thrilled to hear I was rated the most valuable player for our team. With all the great players we had on our team, that was something special. I ended the season with 11 wins and one loss, and had two wins and no losses with one save during the NCAA tournament and College World Series. My ERA was just over 1.00. The All-New England Team named me as one of the starting pitchers, as well. Several other players from our squad were also named All-New England - Tom Michalczyk, Pat Murphy and Don Murelli. Coach V was, of course, Coach of the year. At our banquet, I presented Coach V with an award for passing Springfield College Coach Archie Allen with the most wins in New England. When I made the presentation, I joked to the crowd a little by saying, "Coach V has just passed some guy named Archie." The crowd laughed a bit. Part of life is keeping people happy and smiling.

Now that I got back to Boston, I had to decide what offers I was going to pursue. I had major league tryouts set up with the Chicago Cubs, Kansas City Royals and Milwaukee Brewers. Also, I had another contract with Rome in the Italian Baseball League. And the other two were with the New Brunswick Professional League and the Maine Professional League in Portland.

The first offer I took was in Portland. They offered me living expenses and $200 per game. The first game I pitched, I won 1-0 but it went 12 innings and I went the full twelve. The owner and coach were ecstatic about my showing. The crowds out there loved their baseball. After the game, the owner came up to congratulate me. I told him that if I have to keep working that hard for a win, he's going to have to pay me more money. He agreed. After only the one game, I got a call from New Brunswick and I agreed to a contract with them. This was pretty good but I was still looking for a bigger deal somewhere. I was going to Marysville, New Brunswick. I jumped on a plane to Nova Scotia and someone picked me up at the airport and we drove for about an hour or so to Marysville. I lived with the head coach in a beautiful apartment below where he lived. We had players from all over Canada as well as New England. Our ball club was called the Cosmos. We didn't get our first game started because of a lot of rain for a couple of weeks. The league included a bunch of future major leaguers, including Jeff Reardon, who signed with the New York Mets.

I only stayed with Marysville for a few weeks. I didn't like it much there. I thought I could perform at a higher level. The few games I played in, I pitched very well. In my first game, they pitched a few of us three innings each. I gave up one hit, striking out six. A lefthander we had named

Farnham was pretty good. I followed him after we left but I don't think he got a major league contract with any team but he threw pretty hard; had a great arm. My next game I went about five innings and threw very well again. The head coach used to bring me for lunch and dinner quite often, many times to either Chinese food buffet or dinner. There were chicken farms around the area and he loved chicken. During the day I would go out with some of my teammates. I enjoyed going fishing a lot and did that quite often. The games were at night so keeping busy there wasn't a problem. The coach had a good-looking daughter but she was still a little young for me; but most of her friends were the same age but one girl was a little more my age. I got with her a couple of times but I was bored. I remember the big news around town was a young kid named Paul Hodgson from Marysville who signed with the Toronto Blue Jays. I used to walk down to the corner store and they were talking about him all the time. Later on when I played in the Pioneer League and played against the Medicine Hat Blue Jays, he had just been released from them.

I wanted at this time to push myself to pro ball as best I could. When the major league draft was completed and I wasn't taken, a couple of people said the reason was because my arm had been bothering me and the scouts wanted to see if my arm came around. I was really disappointed because I didn't care how my arm was. I just knew I could get hitters out consistently no matter how my arm was. I knew no one could hit me. Everyone knew that from my record. I knew I could dominate this league in New Brunswick so I wanted to move on with my career.

Bobby Kramer, one of the real nice guys in the game and someone who knows every kid that ever played, is a long-time semi-pro baseball coach who coached Mark "The Bird" Fidrych and many, many more. Bobby paid me an unbelievable compliment. He used to go to far away cities and states to watch me pitch. I never knew him at the time. He would go see me at New Haven and many Intercity League games. He coached for some forty years. He also scouted for the Cleveland Indians. He said, "I've been in this game for forty plus years and Dave is the best I ever saw in this game. He ranks in my top three pitchers of all time with Fidrych and Graig Allegrassa, Fidrych, a great Detroit Tiger, and Allegrassa, a Baltimore Oriole pitcher.

16.

Meeting Elizabeth Taylor, One-On-One

WHEN I RETURNED BACK TO Malden, Trixie was helping me look for work in the hotel field where I had received my degree (hotel management). While I was waiting for hopefully other offers to come through, I started working at the Copley Plaza Hotel in Boston, one of the most elegant hotels in the city. While I was working as a bellman, the Italian League was calling me constantly to offer me a contract. This was going on for a couple of months. We got to the point where I had to go to Bridgeport, Connecticut to meet with them with Coach V, who wanted to be there for the meeting. There were four or five representatives from their league. What an offer. I was going to become the highest paid player ever to play in Italy. They were going to give me $1,200 a week (American money), an apartment overlooking the Coliseum, credit card expenses, a limousine to take me to and from the ball park, all phone call expenses and, last but not least, an opportunity to be in a movie with Anthony Quinn. He was our team owner; the great movie actor. They worked that part of the deal in when they found out my father's past history in Hollywood. I was thrilled, as was my entire family with what was beginning to happen. The other major thing was I was only going to pitch once a week because Rome was only going to play three times a week so pitching once was all I was required to do.

While waiting for all this to happen, I was enjoying working at the Copley Plaza Hotel. Meeting big stars and famous people was enjoyable. People such as Elizabeth Taylor, Pavarotti, Tony Bennett, Ricky Nelson, Yul Brenner, Gina Lollobrigida, Debbie Boone, Burt Reynolds, President Ford,

Natalie Cole, Frank Sinatra, Curt Gowdy, Liza Minnelli, Joan Baez, Bernadette Peters and professional wrestlers, among others.

When the great Frank Sinatra came in town for a week, his secretary had me handling a lot of different requests he and she both needed. I couldn't believe how small a man he actually was. I remember his wife Barbara came in a few hours before he did. When he got to the room, he was really upset with her, angrily stating that she was drinking too much since she had arrived. When he would get off the elevator, it seemed as if it would take ten minutes before you would see him because of all his security people.

Elizabeth Taylor came to Boston a short time later to appear in the play "Private Lives" with her ex-husband Richard Burton. Taylor stayed with us at the Copley Plaza and Richard Burton was staying at the Ritz-Carlton since they were no longer married. Boston was very excited about this play coming to town. Miss Taylor called me down at the concierge desk and asked me to please send out for some movie tapes at Strawberries Music store. I asked her what movies she would like and she only gave me one or two to try to purchase but wanted me to pick out another eight or ten others. It was a Monday and that meant no play at the theater. She said she just wanted to stay in and watch the movies. I sent one of the bellmen out to Newbury Street to purchase them. When he came back to the hotel, I called Miss Taylor's room. When I told her I had the movies, she said for me to come up to the room and she would leave the door open for me. I was pretty excited about seeing her on a one-on-one meeting. When I knocked on the door, she said, "Come in, Dave." When I entered, she was lying on the 500 suite floor in her nightgown. She said, "Sit down and we'll look these over." Looking at her with no makeup on and not dressed to the max made me think "Wow, what a difference clothes and makeup can make for her." She was still attractive but not like what you read about or saw on the screen. I remember looking around while we were on the floor and glancing at the closet. I never saw so many shoes or clothes in all my life. We talked for some time. She asked if I wanted to go to the "evening magazines" big event they were having at Anthony's Pier 4 on the waterfront. She said she was going to invite me. I took my girl Janet Sullivan. She loved Elizabeth Taylor so when I asked her to go, she was ecstatic. When the big night came, Janet was on the dance floor with me and I looked around and Elizabeth Taylor was dancing on my right, Richard Burton on my left, Joan Kennedy was in front of me and James Taylor was behind me. What an event with all these famous people. Janet kept asking me if she could say hello to Elizabeth Taylor. After a short time I said yes and Janet went up to her and spoke with her a few minutes. Someone in my hometown got news of the event and called me and she asked if I slept with Elizabeth Taylor. How stories get exaggerated!

When Gina Lollobrigida came to the hotel, I remember bringing her to her room with the bellman and telling her about my upcoming plans to play in Italy. She smiled and we spoke about how fun it was going to be. She told me how I was going to eat like I've never eaten before. She was very nice but I remember her getting very upset with a few of the girls who were working for her. She had a typical Italian temper. But she was a nice lady. It was enjoyable to see and speak with her. You could tell how attractive she must have been in her younger years.

17.

My Lifelong Dream Comes True

THIS WAS 1978 AND SOME major league teams were in touch with me now. I was gearing up for Italy all this time but once the major leagues were calling, that was always my goal since I was a youngster. The best offer that was coming around was with the Phillies organization. Coach Vieira was now handling everything with the contract. The only thing that seemed to change from day one was now it was a combination of both the Phillies and Seattle Mariners that were to own my contract, but supposedly the Phillies owned a larger portion of it. When we settled in on what was going to happen it turned out I still had to showcase myself in front of the Pioneer League representative where the organization was to be involved. I had to go to New Haven where my alma mater was playing Yale University for the City Series at the Yale Bowl. I was going to perform for them before the game. I stayed in the best shape I could while on my own. This was in May when the Intercity League was beginning its season. The A's were playing against the Hosmer Chiefs and asked me to pitch so I was happy to get in some actual game action before the showcase in Connecticut. I was working out pretty good so I could be ready for the big day in New Haven! Prior to the game against the Hosmer Chiefs, I was starting to feel the discomfort in my right arm again. As everyone who knows me well would attest, I don't complain about injuries or pain. But I was a little worried. When the game came, I was ready. However, the real old juice of my stuff wasn't as sharp as in my previous years. Around the third inning I felt the discomfort again but never said anything to coaches or players and kept battling. We ended up losing the game, one of my few losses in the league over the years. Our left fielder misjudged a fly ball that allowed two runs to score and we lost 3-2 or 4-3. I was mad but I knew it was a tuneup for New Haven. But, I hated to lose nonetheless. There was an old sports article written about me many years ago about how I wasn't like most athletes. It described how I wouldn't accept defeat like most people do. That's why I seldom could lose. I guess I would have taken to the bottle or taken my own life had I lost as consistently as most players did.

When it was time to showcase my ability at the Yale Bowl, my mind was definitely in the right frame but my arm was still bothering me. This particular day, though, I just said to myself, throw as hard as you can. I knew they knew I knew how to pitch. Coach V had been keeping them updated on my past history. They wanted to see me face "live" hitters. So Coach V arranged the hitters to get in the box against me. He put the best hitters in there to face me. The funny thing was Coach, as I found out later, had told the guy watching me (Mr. Nichols) how I had such great control and could put any pitch anywhere I wanted. As it turned out, I couldn't find the plate as I usually could and I hit a couple of the hitters. I was throwing hard, though. The hitters were telling other guys to get in there after they got plunked by me because they didn't want to get hit with another pitch. Trixie was down there with me and he said he had never seen me with that little control. But I threw pretty well anyway. When I finished the workout, my arm was taxed but also sore. When we got back to the university after New Haven won the ball game, they signed me and it finally was over. That was my lifelong dream. Even though I had signed two previous professional contracts in Maine and New Brunswick, this was the big one. From the explanation from Mr. Nichols, my contract was for the Pioneer League with Butte, Montana, and the contract was owned by the Philadelphia Phillies and the Seattle Mariners. They told me the team was going to be managed by Tom Zimmer, son of Boston Red Sox manager Don Zimmer.

In between the time I was negotiating the Italian contract and the time I signed with the Pioneer League, the paperwork with Italy was really getting complicated. But even though the Italy contract would have been the largest ever, I wanted to do what I ultimately did.

Once I signed, the local newspapers, as well as the papers in Connecticut, wrote it up pretty good. There is no feeling like the feeling I had once I signed. It's something like you worked hard all your life for something you love to do and want to do for years to come and you get rewarded. My family was so proud. I remember Rocco and Ann being stopped everywhere they went and being congratulated; Steve and Joan, as well. They were a proud brother and sister, for sure. I remember a few of the guys down Malden Square commenting one day saying, "There's Davey Cai. His brother Steve signed as a pro with the Patriots behind Russ Francis and now brother Dave is a professional baseball player."

Everywhere I would go, people wanted to talk and bartenders and patrons all wanted to send drinks over to me and my friends, even though I wasn't much of a drinker.

The popular North Shore a capella group would invite me on stage to sing with them at local watering holes and introduce me. Richie Willis was the manager and main singer in the group and he was a good friend of mine along with Steve Gambale, Bobby Crowley and Vinny Straccia. All were good guys and they could sing. I was getting so I wanted to be out in the public eye constantly. But at the same time, some people can annoy you, never leaving you alone. Now I was starting to see what Coach Vieira used to say to me many times. He used to say he wanted to stay in more often because no matter where he went, people would bother him and he couldn't enjoy himself. It wasn't to that point yet but I understood what he was saying.

Women from all over were popping up out of the blue to meet me either on their own or through friends or relatives. I was always very cautious, though. I never could determine whether the women were after me because they really liked me or if they wanted to be around an athlete who was well known. My father always said to be careful and make sure you get the right girl. He called them "gold diggers." My brother Steve had a lot of women chasing him around the country so Rocco used to tell him the same thing. He was just being a good father, looking after his kids.

I was to find out shortly that when I got to pro ball everyone was pretty much like I was around these parts. They were exceptional in whatever part of this country or their country they came from. Later on, when we played against the Dodgers' Lethbridge farm club, Jim Lefebvre, the ex-major leaguer and their skipper, told me how he was sure I was the best in my area before signing. But once you get to be a professional, everyone is great. He couldn't have been more accurate.

It was nearing the time in the beginning of June 1978 that I was about to report to Butte, Montana, in the Pioneer League. I was anxious to get started. I knew I could pitch to compete at the next level but I was still constantly thinking of my arm and how severe the injury I was experiencing was. You never want to tell management that you are having arm trouble. So I said I'll go at it 100 percent and see how it holds up.

When I finally got on the plane to head to Butte, so many things were going through my head. Just sitting in the plane thinking of family, friends, the growing up years, etc., that were so important to me made me feel special but sad that I was leaving everything back in Boston. But over the past few years I had been traveling around quite a bit so it wasn't anything new. Just knowing I was going to have highs and lows in the game of baseball was going to be interesting. No one at the professional level ever plays without failures; no one. Even the greatest hitters fail two out of every three at bats, and pitchers with records of sixteen wins and ten losses have completed a so-called good year. That would only be a little higher than a 60 percent winning mark, unacceptable to me in my years up to this point but I knew that would change.

When I arrived in Butte, all everyone heard about was the famous Evel Knievel, the great stunt man/dare devil. He lived in Butte. But he wasn't necessarily in Butte when I arrived. The big story was how he had kidnapped his wife and no one knew where they were. A lot of people in the town did not care for him. As the summer went on, I became friendly with his son Robby. We drove down by his ranch house below the mountains to see where he lived. It was a nice house set alone from other ones. Later in the summer, Evel returned home and was in the Fourth of July Butte parade downtown. From what we heard, people were throwing things at him.

The other thing talked about quite frequently was my relationship with Joe Pepitone. That was in the newspapers quite a bit, as well as the Countrywide Sporting News newspaper. Joe was big; also, playing for the New York Yankees in those days was big time.

18.

Being With Robbie Knievel And Bob Feller

WE WERE WORKING OUT EVERY day getting ready for our home opener against the California Angels Idaho Falls affiliate. Tom Zimmer, our manager, liked what he saw in me. He was a former catcher with the Cardinals. The year before he was a bullpen catcher with the big club. He loved my changeup. He said, "That's the best screwball I ever saw." He compared it to someone on the Cardinals the year before. I told him, "That's my changeup." He said it worked like a screwball. I did turn my change over a bit so that it had that great down and in movement to right-handers and down and away to lefties.

The first game was coming up and I was just getting to know some of the guys. My roommate because we were a co-op team, meaning we had a few affiliates with us, was Hank Bender. He was the number two draft choice of the Seattle Mariners and a catcher. He was from Spokane, Washington. The guys on the team really didn't like him. He acted like he was better than anyone else, and believe me, he wasn't. When we were at home, he was my roomie but, thank God, on the road I roomed with my buddy Ralph Suarez from Philadelphia. Ralph was a lefthanded pitcher and one funny kid. I loved him. He would look out for me like a brother, making sure I stretched out longer than usual before a game, etc.

A few of us pitched in the first game against the Angels, two or three innings each. The first professional hitter I faced was Tom Brunansky. What a monster of a kid he was. I remember throwing a two-seam fastball in on his hands and he muscled it out to deep leftfield that my leftfielder Alvin White caught. Wow, was he strong.

It was good to get my feet wet, so to say. But in the second game of the series something strange happened. One of the Angels players hit a routine ground ball to Julio Franco at shortstop and he threw over to our first base-man Steve Swain. Well, what happened was the runner stepped on Steve's heel. Not knowing if he did it on purpose or not, Swain, after receiving the ball, turned and rifled the ball off the runner's back going up the right field line causing a full-scale brawl. Everyone was fighting, including Zim. He had a pipe in his hand swinging at someone. Was he mad! When the brawl was finally over, I said to myself, "So this is pro baseball!" It looked like it was going to be quite a summer.

After pitching the first game, the pain in my arm was still there. It was like a deadening pain, wasn't sharp but it was concerning. Once again, I wasn't about to tell Zim or Bruce Manno, our general manager, that my arm was giving me trouble. Only the big bonus babies can do that. Because the organization puts in so much money as an investment, they have to treat it as that, an investment. I was beginning to wonder if all the pitching and everyday throwing I did throughout the years might have caught up to me. Zim had me in the starting rotation all along with three other pitchers.

The one major drawback we had as pitchers in Montana was the air. We were a mile high and the air was so thin the ball carried like an airplane. I bet the baseball traveled at least 40 to 50 feet further out there. We always heard stories of how it was pitching in Denver. Now we saw it, first hand.

Zimmer used to tell us that the experts figured to take two or two-and-a-half runs per nine innings and that is what your earned run average should be. Mine by the mid-point in the season was around 5.00 but, with every-thing considered, not bad. I was either second or third on the staff in lowest ERA at that point. Sometimes you would make a great pitch and someone would hit it 400 feet.

Just before one of the games I was pitching against the Calgary Car-dinals, Zim told me the day before to back up Bob Feller in a home run hitting contest. I said, "Who?" Zim said, "Yes, the great Bob Feller." He used to go around to the minor leagues and had five or six guys from either team see if they could hit a home run off him. Well, I was charting that day because I was scheduled to pitch the next day. That's why Zim picked me to feed Feller. When I walked out to the mound I was waiting for his big introduction to the huge sell-out crown. When he walked out, the crowd gave him a thunderous ovation and he loved it. He was a very proud man. I introduced myself to him and he shook my hand. He asked me why the ERAs were so high and I simply told him, "the air up here." The first batter he faced was the Calgary Cardinals manager Johnny Lewis who had just retired from the St. Louis Cardinals the year before. The very first pitch Feller threw him Lewis hit over the 385-foot sign in right. Was Feller pissed! He was mumbling under his breath to me. Later, Lewis hit another one even further, over the 420-foot sign in center. Was Feller ever mad now! He turned to me and said, "No one's ever hit a ball against me like that." This was the great Bob Feller. I didn't know what to say to him but "Bob, I told you, we call this place the airport because balls fly out of here so frequently." He wasn't buying it.

After Feller's performance, I did my running and grabbed my forms to chart the pitchers and hitters for my game the next day. When I went into the clubhouse to shower and get changed to go to the press box, there was Bob Feller showering next to me. I got talking to him a lot. You could tell he was a cocky guy but, as I always go by, if you backed it up, say what you want.

I told him I had heard about how great he was my whole life and how hard he threw. He turned to me and said, "Dave, the thing that used to aggravate me was everyone talking about my fast ball. But he said not only did he have the best fast ball in baseball but his curve ball, as well, that not many people talked about. After he said that, years later Ted Williams said the same thing about Feller's curve ball.

Feller was very nice to me. He asked where I was from and I said Boston. He said his wife loved the Red Sox and if the Sox got into the World Series, he would be behind the Sox dugout. If I got a chance to go, to look for him behind the dugout. As everyone remembers that was the 1978 season when the Red Sox blew a 14-game lead to the Yankees and had the one-game playoff which Bucky Dent won with a home run.

Butte was interesting. I loved the old west from my younger days. We had a few old saloons in downtown Butte we'd frequent. Behind the ballpark was a museum-type configuration of an old western town. It was great to walk through. It had a blacksmith's shop, an old barber shop, a saloon, livery stable, hotel, general store. It was something.

I was really hitting it off with two guys on the team in particular, my road trip roommate Ralph Suarez and my catcher Fla Strawn from Texas. Both were great people. To this day I still talk with them a couple of times a month. Ralph was under the same contract as me being owned by two organizations and Fla was with the Texas Rangers. Ralph kept everybody in stitches on the bench, in the locker room and off the field. Fla was more serious but both were tremendous competitors.

Ralph went on a date with a girl from Butte and it turned out to be some boxer's ex-girl friend. When he heard about Ralph, word got back to us that he was going to shoot Ralph off the mound during a game. If you were outside the ball park, you could see inside from the Montana Tech University building beyond left field. A couple of days later, Ralph was scheduled to make a start. Someone told him he was going to get shot by the guy. Of all days, Zim told me he might need me for an inning out of the pen so I said OK. Sure enough, Ralph gets in trouble in the sixth inning. I was warming up and all of us were eyeing that area beyond the left field wall to see if we saw anyone with a gun. It was difficult to see that far away. A few of the guys in the pen were praying they weren't going to get called in relief of Ralph and be in danger of getting shot off the mound. No one wanted to be within striking distance of Ralph in case a bullet was wide. Well, Ralph started to tire and Zim makes the move with his right hand that he wants me to come in. A couple of the pen guys were teasing me when I left to go to the mound. One said, "Nice knowing you, Cai." As I was walking to the mound, I was hoping Ralph would leave the mound area and begin to walk to the dugout. But Zim had a rule not to leave until the reliever gets to the mound. I really took my time and Zim was signaling me to hurry up. When I got to the mound, Ralph gave me a "Go get 'em, Cai." Then he left. But nothing happened, no gun fire or anything. What a relief!

19.

The Downstairs Disco Near Massacre

NOTHING EVER HAPPENED WITH THE boyfriend and Ralph, and I don't think Ralph saw the girl again. It wasn't anything serious anyway because Ralph really was in love with his girlfriend Denise back home. That's all he talked about, Denise. He was very upset because some guy from the Jersey shore was constantly after Denise. It was the middle of the summer and Ralph knew they would be close by each other. I used to tease Ralph about it. He took it in good humor. He was and still is a wonderful guy. We had some laughs but also some serious moments as well.

Our first trip to Billings to play the Reds was quite an event. Ralph was pitching and my roommate Hank Bender was catching. With the runner on first stealing, Ralph turned slightly too soon to see the throw going down to second. As soon as he turned, the throw from Bender hit Ralph right off the back of the head. They had to take Ralph to the nearest hospital. When he got back to the hotel, he said the doctors suggested not for him to go to sleep or lie down. After we went to dinner, I kept Ralph out until after our curfew and kept giving him a lot of coffee. The next day was my scheduled start. When we boarded the bus, Zim got on the microphone to give out his fines from the previous day. He said, "Fellas, today's starting pitcher Caiazzo missed curfew last night. That's a twenty-five dollar fine." I had told him I had to keep Ralph out and moving, and that was why I missed curfew. He wasn't buying it. Later after the game, he said, "Don't worry about the fine."

That particular game I pitched was against a Reds team that was stacked. It had future major leaguers Skeeter Barnes, Gary Redus, Nick Esasky, Tom Lawless, Les Straker and Charlie Liebrandt.

The first batter I faced was Barnes. He walked to lead off and Redus, who to this day holds the highest professional batting average ever, was at the plate. Barnes was known for his speed. I kept throwing over to first to keep him close. After the fourth throw over, some lady in the front row on the Reds side of the field (first base) kept yelling over "Boring. Boring." She was a nuisance but I kept aggravating her every time I threw over. After about the sixth time I wanted to call my first baseman (Steve Swain) over to let it go so the throw would hit her. But, of course, I wasn't going to do that. But, what a pain in the neck she was.

The game was cruising along around the fifth or sixth inning when Redus came to the plate. He was tearing the cover off the baseball all season, leading the entire league in just about every department. My catcher Fla was calling a pretty good game as he usually did. When we got to a one-ball, one-strike count, Fla called for the fast ball. I threw a pretty good one down in the zone. I couldn't believe what I saw next. Redus crushed it. Sending it deep into the left field area well over the fielder's head. It hit the scoreboard and broke one of the big bulbs for the balls and strikes. I wasn't that upset because I knew I made a good pitch. Sometimes you have to tip your cap to the hitter. He was hitting every pitcher in the league like that, too. When we got through the inning, I got back to the dugout and Zim said, "Where was that pitch?" I said, "Right at his shoe tops." He said, "Are you sure. I told him to ask Fla. Fla said, "Ya, he hit it right off his shoe laces." That was the end of that conversation. Boy, could he hit.

The funny thing was, around the seventh inning, Ralph Suarez came in from the bullpen and when I was sitting in the dugout during our at bat, he said, "Boy, when you give 'em up, you give 'em up." He showed me an area in his arm that got hit by the broken glass and he never let me forget it. Later in the year, Ralph gave up two to Redus in one game and I gave it right back to him.

We lost that ballgame but I was more concerned with my arm again. I just couldn't let my arm come all the way through on my follow through as I could before. Therefore, I had to leave a lot of pitches more in one area, giving the hitters more of an advantage. That area was inside to right-handers. I knew I really had to pinpoint now with my pitches. I couldn't overpower people at all anymore.

When we got back to the hotel there was an attractive girl hanging around our hallway outside our room. I got talking to her and had a nice evening with her. She was one of those girls you knew was looking to find a husband who was going to be making a lot of money in this game. At this time, though, even though I spent a nice night with her, I knew my time in pro baseball was going to be shortened.

After the road trip, when we returned to Butte, I had to see the team trainer about my arm. He sent me to a doctor downtown. The doctor gave me ultrasound treatment and budazolidan pills to take. It was starting to feel a little better as time went on but I was getting a sharper pain if I threw as I had been. What I did was change my arm angle a little bit to compensate for the pain I got.

When we were back, Dad was calling me quite a bit. He was into the astrology, horoscopes, etc. He would call me and ask when I'd be pitching next and how that day was supposed to be for me. I was asking about my Augustine's A's team back home, as well. They were doing well, and Dad said the local papers were following my progress on a regular basis. Evel Knievel's son Robbie was coming around often to where we lived. He loved baseball. He would ask me if I could leave him tickets for our games, so I did. He was a good kid. I did this quite often all summer.

The Toronto Blue Jay farm club, the Medicine Hat Blue Jays, came to play us in a three-game series. After the first night game, some of the guys went downtown to the nightclub known as the Downstairs disco. I didn't go. Ralph, Fla and I went for a local bite to eat, instead. We weren't back from dinner more than ten minutes when some of our guys came running in saying they got in a brawl downtown in the disco with some of the local people from Butte. Gary Ezell and Ronnie Stinnett came back explaining what happened, Some of the Blue Jays players were there, as well, and some of them got beat up pretty badly. Since Butte was known as the toughest town in the United States, some of the locals wanted to prove that, especially to the ball players coming into their town, moving in on their territory. Mike Cuellar, son of the great Baltimore Orioles' lefthander, was a pitcher with Medicine Hat, was at the disco and got beaten pretty badly. He was rushed to the hospital and I remember reading that his Dad had to leave the Orioles to go see him in the hospital. He wasn't at all happy with what happened. Also on that team was a deaf infielder named Montgomery, who also got bloodied pretty good. I really felt bad about that because he couldn't communicate. I remember that when we heard about what happened, we had to go and wake up Zim to inform him. When I spoke with family and friends back in Boston, they said there was a huge article in the Boston Globe about what happened. There was that connection because Tom Zimmer's Dad was Red Sox manager Don Zimmer.

During the home stand, we had a uniform problem. The uniforms we wore at home were our Butte Copper Kings ones. As it turned out, our club house boy Danny while drying them ran into a major problem. He let them go a little too long in the drier and ruined them. Zim had to call the Phillies to get us some of their uniforms sent immediately to us. We were wearing the traditional road powder blue ones but needed those white ones for home games. The uniforms did come in right away and as you looked at them there were some great names on the inside of them. Names such as Jim Lonborg, who I followed as a kid in Boston. He finished up his career with Philadelphia. There was Greg Luzinski and other greats. I wore Wayne Twitchell's uniform, number 33. These were the white with red pinstripes.

20.

Playing With The Great Julio Franco

THE BALL CLUB WAS STRUGGLING. We were at the bottom. We weren't getting consistent pitching or hitting and our defense was shaky most of the games. After a loss, Zim went crazy and called for us to be at the park the next day at noon for a 7:30 p.m. game. He practically ran us into the ground, and it was one of those hot days. All were exhausted. At night when the game was going on, Zim noticed Julio Franco eating a hot dog in the dugout. The girls who worked at the park used to hang out beside the dugout and Julio or any of us would ask them to get us things at times. But, not during a game. When Tom Zimmer saw that, after the game he told us to get to the park early again the very next day. He ran us hard again prior to our regular workout before the game. After the running, he told us he never wanted to see us eat again in the dugout especially during a game.

So the game begins and we're in the second inning and we look over to the end of the dugout and there's Julio Franco eating a hot dog. Three or four of us went over to him and grabbed the hot dog out of his mouth, threw it under the bench and gave him a tongue lashing. Julio was only about sixteen at the time playing professional baseball. You could see that he was going to become exactly what he was as a major leaguer, winning a batting title and become one of the great hitters in the game. He loved his women, and the women loved him, as well. He liked the blonde white girls back then.

My next scheduled start was going to be against the Great Falls Giants. Once again, when I got the start I had to do an event with the clown prince of baseball, Max Patkin. Zim talked to me before I went to the bullpen to warm up. He introduced me to Max as the starting pitcher. What he wanted me to do once I took the mound, I would go through my warmup pitches as usual. Then I was going to put on a great comedy show for the fans, as well as the players. He was funny. When he came to the plate before we started the real game, he wanted me to throw the first pitch a little inside, which I did. He put on an act to get out of the way of the pitch, and he gave me a stare. The next pitch he wanted me to knock him down, which I did, and he got up off the ground and took two steps toward the mound as if he was coming out after me but then he returned to the batter's box. The next pitch he wanted me to throw right down the heart of the plate. When I did, he bunted the ball right down the third base line and legged it out. What a riot! He had that old New York Mets uniform on with a big "?" on the back. He had the crowd in stitches. I was glad I got to be part of the show.

By the seventh inning, we were beating the Giants 2-1 and they had a runner on first base but Patkin was coaching first base for the Giants (all part of the show). But we still had a ball game to win. When I went to pick off the runner, somehow Max got in the way of the first baseman trying to slap the tag on the runner. The ball got loose and the runner ended up on second base. He eventually scored and we were tied going into the last inning. When I was coming back to the dugout after the ninth inning, Max Patkin came running out to greet me in front of our dugout and said, "That a boy, Dave, nice win." I turned to him and said, "Max, we're still tied." He looked at the scoreboard and said, "Oh shit, you're right!" He was a great guy and I was so proud to meet him.

We eventually lost the game but I pitched pretty well. The right arm was killing me but I never said anything and kept taking my pills as the doctor ordered. The arm wasn't getting much better, in fact, it was worse.

21.

"She's A One-night Stand, Not Your Sister"

AFTER THE HOMESTAND, WE HIT the road again, this time to Calgary to play the Cardinals the first night of the series. It was cold there; I'm talking like 30 degrees. It was so cold Zim suggested we get some papers from the concession stand and light two fires in the dugout, one for each barrel that we had. It helped but it was still like New England weather. I wasn't as cold as some of the guys, especially the ones who weren't playing, because I was pitching. I could not get loose once I started throwing in the bullpen. I never got a good feel for the ball.

I went mainly with my curveball in this game because my fast ball just wasn't there. I had to throw a large number of changeups, as well. Fortunately, I had good command of the pitches I was throwing. Otherwise, I would have been lit up. I ran into trouble in the sixth inning and Zim knew I was starting to lose the feel for my breaking ball so he made the pitching change. I left losing by a couple of runs. I didn't give up many but we weren't scoring either.

Tony Jordan, our flame-throwing righthander, pitched the next night and was hit hard. So, I didn't feel too bad but I hate to lose. Ralph Suarez used to tease Tony because he threw so hard. He would get him going by saying, "Tony, once you ring someone up, point him back to the dugout." Tony was such a fruitcake, he listened and used to do it. The bad thing was Tony only had that 96-mile-an-hour fastball with no breaking stuff. So, after the hitters saw him once, they hit him like they owned him. So when he went more than one time through the lineup, it didn't matter how hard he threw, he was in trouble. He could throw but too bad he didn't want to learn to pitch with more of an assortment of pitches. Zim finally caught on to what he was doing by pointing hitters back to the dugout and he knew it was coming from Ralph. He would tell Ralph to stop instigating the situation. Ralph used to make me laugh with that stuff. He was a free spirit himself.

After the game back at the hotel, Tony met some girl from Calgary and we would tease him because he never came out of his hotel room with her. One day we got all over him for bringing her flowers to the room. Ralph used to say, "She's a one-night stand, not your sister."

On the next trip to Medicine Hat, we faced the Blue Jays. Not only did I get my first professional win but I also saw my buddy Fla get beat up behind the plate. The first game we were in it early and Fla got hit with a foul tip and I've never seen anyone in such pain in my life. When he got hit, the training staffs from both teams were out behind home plate taking care of him. After a good ten minutes or so, they brought him into our dugout and into the training room. Man, I could tell that Fla was in so much pain because his face was a different color. The training room and clubhouse was not too far past the dugout so we could hear Fla moaning for a few innings. Wow, did I feel bad for him. Fla was going to be a big loss both on the field with his defense and at the plate, as well. He had so much knowledge of the game. He was great to just sit there with and talk baseball. You would learn an awful lot. Fla was going to miss a couple of weeks with his injury.

The next night I started and what a thrill. To win your first professional game was something. Before the game, I was just unwinding in the clubhouse and we still had plenty of time to go before the game was going to start. I asked Danny, our clubhouse boy, if he could get me something from the concession stand. He said he would but he had to do a couple of things for Zim so I let him take care of that business. I was thirsty so I thought I'd go out to the stand myself. When I got there, a girl was working and I couldn't take my eyes off her. We got talking and she asked where I was from and what position I played. I said, "I'm pitching tonight." She said, "I'll watch you when you're pitching. I'm pretty focused when I pitch but every once in a while I'd look back behind the backstop at the walkway from behind the stands. She was watching every time I looked. I pitched a great game and, boy, did I get support. We won 18-1. Zim took me out after seven innings I remember their two toughest hitters were Brian Milner, their catcher, and Lloyd Moseby, their outfielder who made quite a name for himself for years in the big leagues with the Blue Jays. Moseby had one single off me but I handled him pretty well, and Milner great. Milner was the number two draft pick that year and had it in his contract after he signed to be called up to the big club for a cup of coffee. Well, I guess when he was up there he faced the Orioles. He ended up going something like four-out-of-six in the couple of games he played against Tippy Martinez and Dennis Martinez, two exceptional big league pitchers. I struck out Milner twice in four appearances and he went o-for-four that night. I think I was a little more juiced up for that night seeing Lynda (the concession girl) in the crowd watching me because my arm felt better that night. Also, it was a hell of a lot warmer in Medicine Hat than in Calgary.

Linda met me at the hotel that night and I was so happy to spend some time with her. She was a nice girl, very nice. After the next day at the ballpark, she was so sad to see me leave town and I was sad to leave her, as well. But we stayed in touch every few days. I knew we weren't going back to Medicine Hat again so I was thinking "maybe I won't see this girl again. But then again, I knew I was going to pursue this one. She loved to talk to me on the telephone about how I drove her crazy in my uniform. To be perfectly honest, what drove me to her was when I saw her behind the concession stand in her blue jeans. Wow, was she built well. When I would talk to Lynda on the phone, she would tell me that watching the other players from the other ball clubs coming into town was not the same. That made me feel pretty good. But baseball was my number one priority, not anything else.

Ralph was quite a guy, I was finding out. He was always so concerned with my well-being, making sure I took my insulin on time, that I was eating properly, etc. Ralph was like a real character on and off the field. One game in particular that stands out was when he threw a pitch that the home plate umpire blew a call on. He missed pitch after pitch and Ralph was fed up. When a ball got by the catcher and the runner at third was trying to score, Ralph was covering the plate waiting for the throw from our catcher. When the ump yelled, "He's out!", Ralph responded with "that's right, he's out, and that's where you should be, out!" He then threw the ball completely out of the park We were all laughing to no end on the bench but Zim was furious. He fined Ralph and had him in his office for a meeting about the incident. That wasn't good.

Ralph and I were included in another funny incident. I was pitching and Ralph was in the announcer's booth charting the game. When the announcers asked Ralph what type of guy I was, because he told them we were roomies on the road, Ralph told me he said, "Dave is the nicest guy you'd ever meet anywhere. I love him. Besides that he's the calmest and most unemotional person on the mound but just goes about his business in a professional way. No sooner, he told me, did he say that than I yelled out to the umpire, "Chuck, where was that pitch? I gotta have that one." After he missed a big three-ball, two-strike count that I thought was on the plate, Ralph said you could hear my voice all over the park. He said the announcers for the Idaho Falls Angels faces just dropped. Oh well. I just say that's what happens in the heat of a game. Ralph still teases me about that one.

22.

The Arm Was Getting Very Painful Now

IT'S REALLY AMAZING HOW MANY people follow you once you get into professional ball. We were playing a series in Lethbridge, Canada, against the Dodgers. I was out on the field early doing my work well before the game. Someone signaled me from the third-base dugout area. When I ran in, a guy who was from the New Haven area was following my career and happened to be in Canada and saw that I was in town and came to the game. I never saw him before but that meant a lot to me for him to flag me down to introduce himself to me. He said he used to see me pitch quite a bit when I was at the University of New Haven. He seemed very nice and loved his baseball. He also asked about a few of my old teammates at New Haven and what they were doing now. He also, as everyone usually does, asked about the great Coach Vieira.

The next start I was scheduled for was against the Dodgers. I don't miss those bus trips, sometimes arriving in cities at 7:30 a.m. or 8 a.m., then you have to pitch that day. Not fun. When we arrived in Lethbridge, we almost immediately went right to the hotel restaurant for breakfast. When we sat down at the counter, there was one girl everyone was looking at. She was attractive. Zim was at the counter ordering breakfast himself. Ralph, Fla and I were together a few seats from Zim, who commented on the girl in a positive way. But Ralph commented on how he thought she was looking in my direction a lot. We got talking and I invited her to the next night's game. I was pitching that night. I left her a ticket on the guest sheet. I was geared up pretty good for this start. When I went down to the bullpen to loosen up,

I had to make sure I was stretching out slowly and quite a bit because of my arm. Once I got throwing, I was pretty much finished with about three or four more pitches to go when one of my teammates came running down and said, "Cai, Zim wants you in there." meaning the dugout. I told him, "I'm almost through. I'll be there in a minute or so. I didn't know what he wanted me for, maybe to go over their hitters. I didn't know. Then, just as I approached the front of the dugout, all our players came up onto the front of the dugout because the Canadian and American national anthems were being played. Zim called me to stand next to him. While the American national anthem was being played, he said to me, "Look behind us in the front row. Look who's there." I noticed it was the girl from the hotel restaurant, the girl I left the ticket for.

As it turned out, I threw great that night. I had life in my fastball again and an excellent slider, curveball and changeup. That Dodger team had some great hitters. They had Mike Marshall, the Sax brothers (Steve and Dave), Candy Maldonardo, German Rivera and a kid named Webster, all future major leaguers. I shut them down all night. They were managed by Jim LeFebvre who later made a comment that I threw the best game against them all year. But around the sixth inning, I was facing Marshall, their huge first baseman. He hadn't done anything against me all night. I got to an 0-1 count on him. The next pitch I threw was a curveball and I felt a severe pain in my arm. Marshall swung and missed. But I was in such pain, it was very uncomfortable. I walked off to the back of the mound to let the pain ease a bit. It wasn't going away but neither was I. I wasn't coming off that mound. Fla came out to the mound to ask me what's wrong. I told him, "I'm all right. Go back." The next sign was a fastball. I felt weird. I threw the fastball but Marshall must have thought fastball and it threw him off. He was way out in front of the pitch. I was thinking so much of the pain I couldn't get enough arm speed to throw it hard. Marshall popped up the pitch and I went into the dugout, that being the third out. When I got into the dugout, Zim asked me what was wrong. I told him I hurt something on the next-to-last pitch. He wanted to take me out but I said, "No. I'm going back out." After our half inning, I took the mound. When I threw my first warmup pitch, it reached halfway to the plate. It hurt like hell. The next pitch I threw landed even closer to me than the catcher. That was it. Zim took me out and I was out of action for a couple of weeks.

I saw the Dodgers trainer. Then I saw our team doctor when we got back to Butte. I was really depressed after the game after pitching so well. It was getting to be where I hated to perform at the level I was performing at even though I was still pitching pretty well. I just couldn't make my pitches to the spots I used to and throw with the degree of consistency I always had before. It was frustrating not being able to go out to the mound as I had been every four or five days.

I always looked back and said those $500,000 bonus babies could tell the organization when they're hurt and they are kept on the disabled list until they're ready to come back, whereas the guys who didn't get that type of money either couldn't say anything, like myself, or if they did say they had an injury, they were let go. But by pitching hurt for that long a period of time, I was only damaging the arm even more.

Lynda from Medicine Hat was calling quite a bit and we were in touch. But I still had to deal with the girl, Maureen, from the Lethbridge restaurant. After the game in which I hurt my arm badly, she waited for me outside the clubhouse and we made arrangements to meet back at our hotel. Ralph knew what was going on and offered to sleep in one of the other rooms so I could be with Maureen. That's what your teammates are supposed to do for each other. I did it for my roommates plenty of times over the years.

Zim had seen Maureen with me in the lobby that evening and someone must have told him we were going upstairs. When we got to my room, we had something to eat and watched some television. Within no time, though, we were having sex. But I remember being really low with my blood sugar count and I was tired, really tired. When she was lying on top of me, I heard voices. I didn't think much of it but then Maureen said to me, "What was that?" I said "What?" She turned behind her and could hear people talking almost right outside the room. My room was on the third floor. When I glanced behind her, I saw Tony Jordan's head looking through the window into the room. I couldn't believe what I saw. I guess Zim had organized this by getting a ladder and some of the guys to help get Tony on the ladder and looking through the window. Next thing I heard was a siren from a police car. I could hear Zim yelling for Tony to get off the ladder and for everyone to get out of there. He must have thought the police were coming after him. I don't know. What a scene. I told Maureen she must have been dreaming or something but there was no one at the window. She bought it. When she finally left around 1 a.m., I walked her downstairs to the lobby and, sure enough, there was Ralph lying down on the lobby couch. What a night and day this was. My mind was back on my physical health again.

We got back to Butte after the long road trip. The team was stuck in last place and Tommy Zimmer wasn't happy. He got thrown out of so many games for arguments with umpires that we were all amazed. He had a temper like his dad's. I knew I wasn't going to be pitching in the next homestand for sure. I was just rehabbing. The team doctor was giving me ultrasound, cortisone and I was still taking my pills.

Our homestand wasn't much better than how we had been playing all season. After about a week's rest, I began to throw lightly in the pen before games. The arm wasn't good; I knew that. Each session I threw, I told Zim the arm was getting better but it wasn't. When I was ready to pitch again, it was going to be on the road against the Helena Phillies. It was a double-header and I was scheduled for the second game. I was priming myself for this for some time. When the day finally came, I was anxious to get back out on the field. Our starting pitcher in the first game was Mario Mudano, a lefthander we acquired from the San Diego Padres. He had a rubber arm. He pitched pretty well. Around the seventh inning, it started to get really cold. Zim came down to where I was sitting in the dugout and said, "You're not going to pitch the second game; you'll pitch in a couple of days." I was really mad. Ralph told me to relax and not get upset. But I almost went after Zim. Ralph had to hold me back. I was sorry I got so mad because later I realized he wasn't pitching me because it was cold and I'm sure he didn't want me to reinjure my arm. He was right.

When we were in our hotel in Helena, I was going down to the lobby by elevator to get a sandwich. When the elevator doors opened on one of the floors, in came famous sportswriter Bob Ryan. I thought I recognized him but I didn't say anything. He must have known I was a ballplayer and asked me where Tom Zimmer and Dave Caiazzo were. I said, "I'm Dave Caiazzo." He introduced himself and said the Boston paper sent him out to do a story on us. He asked about the famous fight in the disco in Butte. As I said earlier, we got a lot of exposure because of that. I told Bob Ryan what room Zim was in and he went to catch up with him.

As much as the road trips were fun, I hated to take those long, ten-to-twelve-hour bus rides more than anything. Not only that, we had a bus driver, the same one all the time, named Sean. The guy used to drive us crazy more than anything. The guy would fall asleep while driving in the early morning hours when it was still pitch black outside. We used to have one of us stay awake to keep him awake. Also, on those bus trips, some of the guys would sleep in the overhead luggage bins rather than in the regular seats. Tony Jordan would always drink milk. It seemed he had a quart of milk with him everywhere he went. Sometimes he would take it to the luggage bin with him and when he would fall asleep, the milk would always tip over and spill on someone. That almost started a few fights on the bus.

The Dominican players loved their music and would put their boom boxes up very high. You couldn't sleep at times. Zim would come back from his seat and say, "Shut that fuckin' music off." He didn't like that stuff. He did, however, like Richard Prior. He would put his tapes on so we could all get a few laughs. The big music at this time was John Travolta and Grease. Guys would be playing that constantly on the bus trips and in the locker room.

I was still trying to stay on top of my diet because of my diabetes. That was always tough, especially when we were traveling. Sometimes you would be at the park for six to eight hours, or longer. Then, if you hit the road after the last home game, you left as soon as the game ended. I had to make sure I had food handy all the time. My normal eating regimen was always changing. Earlier in the summer, the weather was much warmer so I would burn off a lot of calories very quickly. That was extremely difficult to control. Sometimes the young girls working at the park would come by and ask me if I needed any food at the concession stand. A couple of them knew I had diabetes, so that helped. One game early in the season I honestly thought I was going to pass out just doing my workouts before the game. I really think the only two guys who knew how bad I was doing with my diabetes at times were Ralph and Fla. They were great, great guys, always watching over me.

23.

Named "Athlete Of The Decade" For The '70s

I CALLED HOME TO MALDEN one night and asked Dad how my old Augustine's A's were doing in the playoffs and he said they just got beat in seven games by the Wakefield Merchants. Wakefield was run by Les DeMarco, a longtime coach and former player. He was one of the great guys you run into in this game that you just like, very personable and easy to talk to. Russ, from home also mentioned that the local newspaper put an article in the paper saying something to the effect that "if Dave Caiazzo was in an A's uniform, there's no doubt the A's would have won that championship series."

It was 1980 and a decade of much success had just ended. What wasn't expected was that the local newspapers were coming up with an "Athlete of the Decade" award from the Malden-Medford area. Paul Leahy, the local sportswriter, called me one day and said they had decided to select me for that award. I was very appreciative. There were many pretty good athletes to choose from. The one I remember was a kid from Malden named Matty Marden. He was a great hockey player from Malden High who went on to play hockey at Boston University when they won the national title. That was a very nice award to receive. Paul had written about consistency and dominance throughout the 1970s. The article was a full front of the sports page.

I finally made my return to action with a pitching start after a long layoff. I threw all right but tired a bit in the late innings. Once again, my focus was in keeping the ball down, moving it around and hitting my spots. The strictly fast ball days were over. I knew it now; it was becoming more evident to me. The one thing I knew I could do better than anyone anywhere was "pitch." No one could pitch better than me. Everyone who saw me pitch over the years would tell you that.

Even though I wasn't pitching up to my standards, I was still proud of how and what I did between the lines and the arm I was now pitching with. One of my teammates said, "Most people would have walked away if they had to deal with what you have to deal with." But my father Rocco brought us up to be men and not be babies. Be tough.

The season was now winding down. It was getting cold after the sun would go down. So many nights we'd have to put on two coats in the dugout, and especially in the bullpen where it was wide open.

A lot of the people we had become friendly with throughout our season were people we may never see again in our lifetimes. The Dougans were a family we all loved. They were real baseball fans who had season's tickets to all our games and even made some road trips. They had us to their trailer park home once every home series began. They were wonderful people. Jim, the husband, and Ginny, the wife, knew every player in the league. The only person on our team they weren't fond of was Hank Bender. Not many people took to him. One time he hit a home run and the home fans at our ballpark started to boo him. He ran around the bases as fast as he could then, when he got to home plate, he flipped the crowd the bird. The boos got even louder. What a jerk he was. I don't know how I lived with him most of the year. Ralph and I ended up living together at home at the end of the season. Years after playing in Butte, Jim and Ginny stayed in touch with me. But about twenty years later, Ginny called me in Boston crying. It was pretty late at night. She told me Jim had died. I felt terrible. I think they had split up for the last couple of years. I think Jim had started to drink and I think he died in a driving accident. What a shame. People couldn't believe how long they stayed in touch with me after the year we met.

The game of baseball brings to you many outstanding people. I learned that back in the day anyway, you stay out of trouble with athletes, for the most part. There are some who aren't your normal good people. Many times I would sit in my room or in my car or anywhere and think how lucky I was to have what I have, and have accomplished what I had. The more I looked at some families, the more I appreciated mine.

Steve had been back now from Toronto in the Canadian Football League. He just couldn't stand on that knee any more. It really was a shame his career fell short. As I was starting to see, injuries are a big part of whether someone makes it big or not. I always said, "You have to be lucky and stay injury free." Steve had more talent than anyone I had seen in my day. Eddie Rideout, who I had played baseball against but whose main sport was football, was the other person who I thought had unbelievable talent. Eddie turned out to be a close friend of mine and my brother's. He was a Boston College grad who was drafted by the Boston Patriots. He was electrifying on the football field as a wide receiver and punt and kickoff return man.

Now that the season was closing down, I looked back and said that I think I got the most out of what I had left. I battled and kept my injury for the most part quiet. Fla, my catcher, used to say, "I knew you were hurting but I knew you could pitch." That alone was a compliment. He knew about pitching but I got a kick out of him when he'd come to the mound saying "I'll take full responsibility for anything I call behind the plate." He could catch!

The guys like Ralph, Fla and even Greg Moore, the big righthander from California, were going to be missed. Moore was about 6 foot, 6 inches tall. He was a good kid out of high school. I'll never forget, before games when we were taking batting practice or infield, he would somehow sneak up to the public address system and turn on the mike before anyone was in that area. He would get on the mike so everyone on the field could hear, "Big Dave, wheelin' and dealin'." The guys used to get a kick out of that. He was such a big kid with a great personality. But he had that competitiveness in him. I was going to miss him almost as much as Ralph and Fla. I really liked Tom Zimmer, as well. He treated me like a man, not a kid; never talked negatively to me or treated me with disrespect. But he expected you to play hard for him. That I did, and I think that's why he had me in the starting rotation all season. I got along with him pretty much all season with the exception of the one time in Helena, but he was a good person, as was his wife, Marian.

I knew Zim had to fill out daily reports directly to the organization after the games. So I knew they were made aware of my arm injury. That I felt uncomfortable with but that's the way it was. I couldn't do anything about it. So whether I was going to come back the next year was up to the organization and whatever General Manager Bruce Manno thought about the future with each individual on the team. It was going to be a business decision and we all knew that. At this point I just wanted to get my last start in and get ready to head home. The entire team was thinking about getting back to their homes, wherever that was.

What you find, by playing ball with all kinds of people from different countries is how you jell with people. In college, I played with whites, blacks, Portuguese, whatever. Once you play professionally, you play with blacks, whites, Dominicans, Koreans, Venezuelans, etc. You live with these guys day in and day out, you eat breakfast, lunch, dinner and sleep in the same room with them. So you have to bond with them. Some you do and others you don't. I got along with pretty much everyone. You knew that this experience wasn't coming around again in your lifetime so make the best of it.

About a week or so before the season ended, Mom and Dad sent me one of their care packages from Malden. It included cookies, crackers, prunes, pepperoni, cheeses, newspaper articles and a bunch of other things. Ralph would always sneak in to grab some food. He loved those goodies. I would miss those packages but knew I was heading home soon for home-cooked meals from Mom and Dad. Steve and Joan could cook, as well.

Lynda was still in touch quite often but Maureen and a bunch of the other girls I went out with or saw on a road trip were just short-lived acquaintances.

After our final game, we all headed home in different directions. Ralph and I, however, went in the same direction. Ralph is from Philly so we flew into New York together. When we separated, we both had tears in our eyes. But we knew we would both soon see each other again. We experienced an unforgettable summer and the friendship we developed was more important. The same went for Fla; we would be buddies forever.

When I got home, I couldn't help but continually think of how I could have prevented my arm injury. So many times I could have said "no" when asked to pitch; days when my arm was sore or taxed, or even when I might have had a slight hamstring pull or something like that. But I wanted to compete constantly. I just knew that even if I was 75 percent healthy, I was better than whoever I was facing, no matter how good he was. So I have no second thoughts on that, especially if I knew it was a big game and I would have cheated my team if we had to throw someone on the mound who may not have been that good. Taking good care of myself was especially important and I did that. Imagine had I not, what the results would have been.

Now I was just waiting to see what would happen with the organization. They knew my arm was pretty much gone; getting cortisone, ultra sound and taking budazolidan tablets wasn't helping. They knew that as well as I did. I was expecting the worst.

24.

Couldn't Dominate Diabetes Like I Could Hitters

IT WAS GOOD BEING HOME with the family and friends again. Some friends, not necessarily close ones, would want to go out a lot. I think just so they could get attention from people. No matter where I was or what we were doing, people would send over drinks or comp a meal or do something for me. That was nice but my close friends wouldn't do that. They knew I liked the attention but sometimes I just wanted to low key it. The attention wasn't something I craved now. The local Babe Ruth League in Malden had asked me to speak at their banquet in October. Johnny Pesky, the great Red Sox player, manager, coach and long-time icon, was the guest speaker and I was the other speaker. Pearl Verge, who I knew for years, asked me if I would speak. Pearl was the mother of one of Steve and my good friends when we were growing up in our neighborhood. She was a very nice lady. She did a lot for the league. The first thing I asked Pearl was if I could invite Rocco and Ann to the banquet. She said "of course." When they introduced me, I spoke about growing up in Malden and playing in the league when I was younger. Also, I spoke about pro ball and what it expects from each player and coach. The most important part of my speech was introducing Mom and Dad. I asked them to stand. They received a great ovation. I was so proud, as I'm sure they were. What I mentioned was how important they had been to me in my lifetime and the sacrifices they made so their kids could lead a better life. I said, "Not only did they develop one professional athlete, but two. Not too often do you see sons sign contracts in two different sports."

Many of the kids and parents were asking for autographs. It was fun. Autographs were always nice to do but some people abuse it. In the minors, I remember we couldn't sign for anyone once the National Anthem was played. One time before game time, people were above our dugout hanging their game programs over the edge to be signed. We would come out of the dugout so they would know who was signing the programs but if you looked at them, you could see the programs already had some names three or four times.

David Jamieson, my boss at the Copley Plaza hotel, had asked me to come back to work. I did. It was something I enjoyed doing. Plus, that was my major in college, hotel management and administration. At one point, Dave had me on the schedule thirty-eight consecutive days. Whenever I was off a day or so, he would call me in to work. He used to say he loved working with me. That's always nice to hear from your boss.

Trixie and I got talking and we decided to get away on a cruise to the Caribbean on the Carnival cruise ship out of Miami. It was an amazing eight-day cruise to San Juan, Nassau and St. Thomas. We met some nice people on the boat. Trixie had everyone laughing throughout the cruise. One day in particular, the ship couldn't dock in St. Thomas because of a tropical storm. It was announced that free drinks would be served for two hours. I wasn't much of a drinker but I said "why not." I had two Kahlua sombreros. They were very strong. I drank them down like I was drinking a glass of water, very fast. This day was very sunny and hot. When we did our regular daily things, nothing seemed different and I felt, pretty good. The main thing back in those days was I never ever checked my blood sugar level. By having those two drinks, I'm sure it went way up to 400 or so. The next morning when I got up, I was disoriented. When you get extremely high one day, the next you get extremely low. I bet I was at 30 on the blood sugar level. We decided to eat breakfast but I probably gave too much insulin and didn't have enough food so my level was still very low.

After Trixie and I ate, we decided to up to the top of the ship to get some sun. It was very hot that day. I remember there were about ten of us sitting together. After a short time, I felt like I was going to die. I was dehydrated and thirsty to no end. After a short time, I couldn't remember anything else. I woke up in the ship's hospital ward. Trixie told me I had collapsed and fallen from the lounge chair and the people couldn't wake me up. Trixie said he was nervous. They called the ship's purser's office and I was carried by stretcher to the hospital ward. What I do remember is not being able to talk at all. My mind basically wasn't functioning properly. Trixie told me the girls we hung out with a lot on the cruise wanted to go visit me, so everyone was at my bedside. Trix said I wasn't talking at all. He told the nurses I was a pro ball player and asked me to sign an autograph for each of them. I don't recall any of that. He said I basically wrote a straight line for my autograph so he said he knew I was messed up.

I remained in the hospital ward until the night before we were to arrive in Miami. I wasn't the same guy. I knew it and Trix and everyone else saw it, as well. I really couldn't communicate well. Trix was saying on the plane from Miami to Boston that I wasn't talking much. When we got back home, I went right back to work at the Copley. After two work days, I called my Dad to pick me up and take me to the hospital. I was kept overnight but they couldn't give me an accurate answer to what was happening to me.

After a month or so, I started to feel better and more like myself. Slowly but surely I got back to normal but one morning I got a call from Marge Candito, the University of New Haven athletic department secretary. I was so low with my blood sugar that I was basically not even talking to her. She would ask me questions and she got no response. She was very concerned and called back at my house to speak with my Dad and he came in to give me some orange juice. I think he gave me two glasses. I was that bad.

As bad as this diabetes was, I was glad I had it and not some young kid. I didn't want anyone to have to deal with what I was going through morning, noon and night. Not one day was going by when I felt good throughout the entire day but I did know there were many youngsters who had the disease.

25.

Helping Future Cy Young Award-Winner Steve Bedrosian

AS I WAS STARTING TO prepare myself for the rest of my life, many opportunities came my way and many things came to my mind. One politician in Malden stopped me on the street in Malden Square. He and I spoke for quite a while. I told him I still wasn't sure what was going to happen to my baseball career at this time. He said, "Dave, don't forget you're part of the most famous family in Malden. If baseball doesn't work out, something else will." I never forgot that and worked hard at no matter what I did. I never wanted to give the Caiazzo family a bad name. One thought I had was to get into coaching.

A few months later, the biggest disappointment in my life had come. I got released. All the years someone puts into the game and then one day, it's over. My arm just couldn't come around. The local sportswriter asked me about the arm and I put it simply, "It's like losing your best friend."

Now I knew I had to pursue another path in life. Someone had called me about the Suffolk University baseball coaching becoming available. I applied and had some great references. This took some time and I was in touch with the athletic director constantly. He did say to me that they had more than fifty applicants and they narrowed it down to myself and Red Sox reliever Jim Willoughby. They finally gave it to him. From what I heard, his wife worked in the office at Suffolk. So, it didn't surprise me but

I was disappointed. It was a Division Three program but I figured I could build their program. But it wasn't going to happen.

My next thought was to start a baseball camp. Ron Luongo, the righthander from Everett who was on the other side of the field when I struck out twenty batters, was just released by the Yankees. We got talking and began the Greater Boston Baseball Camp. The first year we did well but it was only the first year. The only other baseball camp in the Boston area was the Ted Williams Baseball Camp down toward the Cape and the Mike Andrews Camp. Ron only did it for two years and then went into the jewelry business. I really got it going the next year and renamed it the Dave Caiazzo Baseball Camp. We were getting a lot of kids. One of the kids we had was Dana Rosenblatt, who went on to become New England boxing champion. He was a pleasure to work with. Let me tell you, he loved baseball. Loved it! His father Steve and his mother Harriett were wonderful people. Harriett was a riot. She would always try to marry me off. She introduced me to a couple of women I dated. Both were very nice but I just wasn't ready to get serious. Years later, she would tease me about getting married some day. Steve, Dana's dad, was always down watching me pitch for the A's at Devir Park even before I knew him. Nice man.

While contemplating my future plans, Dave Jamieson at the Copley Plaza hotel kept giving me better jobs. Quickly I went from bellman to doorman to bell captain to concierge. When Dave finally offered me the concierge position, I accepted. That was a great job. Dave was the head of our department. There was me and Jim Carey. Jim was the guy I got the job for originally! He was a nice kid. We had a lot of fun on that job.

Jim and I met a few women, to say the least, while at the hotel. One girl I met was with a friend who Jim liked. After we would finish work at night, we would go out to eat somewhere close by. They were from Ohio. Jim loved the famous people who would come to the hotel. He looked forward to that more than anything. He was fun to work with.

My sister Joan was now starting to act a bit out of the ordinary. We were getting concerned with her. She was becoming very friendly with some strange people, which was out of the ordinary. Rocco and Angeline were starting to notice some strange things happening, as did Steve and I. One incident in particular that disturbed me was when I came home one day to find some strange faces in our house. Dad and Mom both were working and Steve and I were out of the house but when I came home I saw these faces I had never seen before. My Italian temper kind of kicked in and I threw them out of the house. A few weeks after that, I looked in my drawer and noticed jewelry and money missing. I hit the roof and exploded on

Joan because we knew it was the people she had let into the house. But Joan was still a little off with the way she was talking and acting. Rocco and Ann decided to take Joan to a doctor to get checked out. The diagnosis was she needed lithium in her body. We were told at the time it was a chemical imbalance. A more modern medical term now would be bipolar. It's a state of depression and, like me with my medication for diabetes, she couldn't be in a normal state without the lithium. She was basically welcoming any type of person into her life. She would just meet someone on the street and act like she knew them for years. But we all knew whatever was happening wasn't her fault. It was a serious situation. As she was taking this medication, it was starting to work. At times she would need to get it adjusted, though. It was always a work in progress but she was starting to improve. That's all the family wanted, to see her healthy.

Coach V asked me to help coach the pitchers down in Daytona Beach during spring training. So, I did that. I figured it would only help somewhere down the line plus I enjoyed working with and teaching kids. One of the prize kids I was working with was future Cy Young Award-winner Steve Bedrosian. We nicknamed him "Bedrock," a name that stayed with him throughout his major league career. I remember getting to the field one day and Coach V pulling me aside. He said, "Cai, take Bedrosian and work with him especially on the slider." Man, could Bedrosian throw. He had an arm most people dream of having. He just loved to throw. As a matter of fact, I used to tell him to sit down and not throw so much. I figured he would end up injuring his arm somewhere down the road. We gave him the nickname because he loved to mix it up a bit. The guys told me that during the school year he punched out a few guys. So we called him "Rocky" after the movie and added "Bed" like the beginning of his name.

I worked with him on his slider and some of his mechanics. He never forgot it. After the season, he got drafted by the Atlanta Braves in the third round. When he made it to Triple A Richmond, there was a huge article in one of the big newspapers. Steve called to tell me he mentioned me in the article. He said how I was the one responsible for helping him with his slider. A couple of years later, he got married and asked me to be in his wedding party. It was in Spartansburg, South Carolina. What an event that was. Steve, of course, was now a major force on the Braves' pitching staff. Also in that wedding were guys such as Terry Forster, Joe Cowley, Matt Sinatro, Ken Oberkfell and Jerry Royster. Steve's wife Tammy had some great-looking girlfriends there, as well. One was a girl named Annie and a girl named Bobbi Eakes, who was Miss Georgia. Annie and I got along well. Steve said she would always ask for me years later but I never pursued it.

The night before the wedding we were in the hotel lounge after rehearsal practice and found out that Bedrock punched out a guy on the elevator. Steve said the guy said something negative about some piece of clothing from Boston he was wearing and they got into an argument. After knowing Steve for only a couple of years, that was a very special thing he did, extending himself for me. I know he respected me but he also appreciated me helping him. We all became pretty good friends from the wedding. Steve also invited Trixie as a guest. He got to know Trixie because Trix used to attend the weekend games at New Haven a lot.

It was now 1983 and my brother Steve and I decided to open a sports bar and restaurant. We took over the famous Tricca's restaurant on Pearl Street in Malden. It was in a residential neighborhood. We built the business pretty well and we started to get some pretty famous athletes to visit. We named it Caiazzo's Playoff Pub. People such as Jim Nance, the great running back for the Boston Patriots came in; John Kennedy of the Red Sox, Bedrock came in a few times.

When the New York Yankees were in town, I would pick up Joe Cowley (from Bedrock's wedding) and he would bring his friend, pitcher Ed Whitson. When Julio Franco came into town, I would get him to come in. After a couple of years, Andy Brickley, who I played baseball with, was now with the Boston Bruins and he would bring the whole team down. Steve Cai became very good friends with Lyndon Byers, Cam Neely and Rick Middleton. Andy Brickley's brother, John, who I was close with, worked my baseball camp for a number of years. Very respectable family.

Cowley was with the Yankees for two seasons, 1984 and 1985. He was a pretty good one, as well. He was 9-2 and 12-6 in those two years. The next year he threw a no-hitter for the Chicago White Sox against the Los Angeles Angels. A night after he and Ed Whitson (one of the other Yankee starters) were at my Pub in Malden. They were drinking pretty good and having a good, old time.. They wanted to close our place. All night long I would say, "Let's get you guys back to the Sheraton. You're probably going to get fined for missing curfew." They kept saying, "We're all right." Around 1 a.m., I got them both in my car and was driving them back. Joe kept saying to Eddie, "We're going to catch hell from Billy." Billy was, of course, manager Billy Martin. Ed was saying, "Don't worry about him. He's probably out drinking himself." Once I pulled up to the front door of the Sheraton, I said, "Thanks for coming, guys, and I'll see you both at the ballpark before the game." No sooner did I say that when Joe said, "Stay in the car, there's Billy." As we looked up, there was Billy Martin stumbling trying to get in the revolving door. Joe said, "Cai, he's like this almost every night."

Eddie wasn't hitting it off with Billy or the Yankees. He was under a huge contract and wasn't living up to what they expected. He was telling me that when the Yanks got back to New York, he was calling his agent to get him out of New York City. He wanted to go back, if possible, to San Diego or Los Angeles. The next stop for them was Baltimore. What happened next in Baltimore wasn't good. While in the hotel hallway, Eddie and Billy got in an argument and Eddie broke Billy's arm. Next thing you knew, Eddie was traded to San Diego.

The Pub was the biggest thing in town. Rocco would do a lot of running errands, keeping the place clean, etc. He would never stop. We used to try to slow him down but you couldn't do that with him. He wanted the best for his boys and he was a stubborn Italian. He would even pick up the debris on the streets to keep them clean.

Because of all the activity from the bar, the neighbors were beginning to complain. We couldn't help the business activity problem. We weren't going to tell people not to come in because the neighbors were complaining. But we did the best we could while monitoring the parking and outside noise as best we could. We used Chris Fallon as our attorney. Chris was a good guy. At one point we had to meet with the liquor board at City Hall in front of the neighbors. Steve got up to speak and when one of the neighbors gave a false statement, Dad started to make his way to the microphone. Chris quickly intercepted Dad's progress and we got him to sit down. He was angry at some of the statements being made. He was a very proud man and only told the truth. He couldn't understand this. Chris did very well for us and they didn't close us for a period of time.

But as the time went on, the Pub was getting to be a headache. It was starting to disrupt our family and it just took up too much of our time. Steve had now left his job at the Correction Department and I was still working at the hotel. Some of the characters the bar attracted were out of a horror movie. We had doormen working but some of the time Steve and I would have to break up fights, etc. We found out a lot of times the girls would instigate the problem and then the guys would be fighting one another and, of course, the girls get out of the way.

I stayed in the business for a few years and then realized that Steve and I were not as we used to be as brothers because of the business. A lot of the patrons would take sides and then Steve and I realized this. We used to talk and Steve would say to me, "You don't think I care about this guy or that guy, do you?" Then I realized he knew a lot of these people were just short-time acquaintances and not family. I got out of the business basically because my brother meant more to me than an acquaintance.

When Steve and I were having problems, someone came into the Pub and went up to him. The guy started to ask about what was going on with us. Steve grabbed him by the neck and threw him out. Someone told me Steve said to the guy, "Don't you ever question anything about me and my brother. He's my brother!" That was good to hear. People, especially in bars, like to gossip. They have nothing else to do while they're drinking.

Toward the end of my time before I left the bar, I started to date a girl named Sheri. I met her coincidently when I was at the Palace nightclub. Jim Carey went up to her and asked where she was from. When she said, "Malden," Jim responded, "Do you know Dave Caiazzo?" She said something like "I think so." Jim said, "I'm with him now. Let me get him." When I went to meet her, she was nothing less than striking. We talked and she gave me her telephone number and we began to date. I even put her on as a barmaid at the Pub. When Coach V came to the Pub to visit me, I introduced Sheri and he just adored her. As a matter of fact, he would come to visit more often just to see her. He would come to Sheri's house in Medford to visit her. Coach had that eye. She was not only a great girl but I was really attracted to her. She would come down to my semi-pro A's games and my teammates would go crazy looking at her. She was a sexy woman. One of my teammates, John Carco, a good friend of mine, asked me if I wanted to do some photographing and modeling with her. But we said no to that. I know he was disappointed. Once I met Sheri's mother, I knew Sheri couldn't have been an unattractive girl because her mother was also very attractive, and nice as well.

The only problem I had with Sheri was that she was a single mother. She had a son who was only about one year old when I met her. Coach V used to take him for walks. But I wasn't ready for a family yet so I started to drift away gradually. I could never say anything bad about her. We got along great. It was just at that time I wasn't ready for a family. Maybe some time soon but not at this time.

One of my teammates in those years used to comment, "She looks amazing in those jeans." Sheri and I reached an understanding not to date any longer. We remained good friends after that. The person most upset with the breakup was Coach V.

Now that I got out of the restaurant business, I was pursuing other interests. The baseball camp was going very well. I had great instructors and the community and surrounding cities and towns were sending me a lot of kids. The instructors I hired were people such as Joe DiSarcina, John Brickley, Bob Ware (a very good baseball coach and friend), Billy Ryan, Bobby Guidi, Chris Nance, Ernie Ardolino, and people like that. I only wanted good baseball people not just anyone. Coach V. would also make appearances. What an impact he made. Arthur Hartung also was helping. He was a former farm hand with the Brooklyn Dodgers and the Cleveland Indians. The local newspapers, the Malden Evening News and the Medford Mercury, gave me great coverage.

One of the kids I had at the camp since he was nine years old was a boy named Rich Barker. He attended the camp for years but then also used to come to me for private pitching lessons. He was talented. When he was older, he signed with the Chicago Cubs and eventually made it to the big leagues. Another local boy was Kevin McGlinchey. He lived right down the street from me. His mother and dad used to come into the Pub. Barbara would always show a great interest in Kevin, as did his dad, Freddy. Kevin eventually made it to the major leagues with the Atlanta Braves.

Andy Brickley used to come down to talk with the campers and sign autographs. He was great. What a great kid! Before I would introduce Andy to the kids and parents, I mentioned how he actually liked baseball better than hockey. He would tell great stories of the Bruins and a lot of the kids were Boston Bruins fans so they enjoyed the talk.

26.

My Friendship With Rico Petrocelli

NOW THAT MY NAME WAS out there quite a bit, organizations would ask me to put on clinics indoors in the winter or clinics during the summer.

Rico Petrocelli, former great Red Sox shortstop, one day called me asking me to help him with his camp. He got my telephone number from someone who knew me. Rico was a guy I immediately bonded with. When we got talking, I mentioned I was related to Joe Pepitone. Rico and Joe had a famous altercation in a Red Sox-Yankees game years ago. I asked Rico about the fight and he downplayed it. He said they were just joking. He said they couldn't fight one another because their noses were too big to get that close to each other. Rico always had, and still does have, a great sense of humor.

He turned out to be someone I deeply respected and I would sacrifice anything for him. He is that nice a person; not only Rico but also his wife Elsie and children. He's a great role model.

Rico would come to the camp, as well, and work with each kid individually, sign pictures, give out gifts and make a great speech each year. When he would leave the park, I had to chase him down to give him some money for doing what he did. That was the hardest part, try to get him to take the check. He would run off into his truck and I would sprint toward the truck and he would lock the door or close the window so I couldn't give it to him. Most of the time he just wouldn't take it. Even though we were friends, I still felt that he went over and above to do me this favor.

When I began to give pitching lessons, Rico and I worked side-by-side a lot in the cages indoors. One funny story about Rico: He was working on hitting with two young boys in the cage to my right, I was working with a couple of kids on pitching. One of the fathers happened to say something to one of the boys in Rico's cage and Rico didn't like it. Rico didn't disrespect anyone but whatever the guy said, it got Rico very upset. He started to go in the direction of the guy. When I saw he was losing his temper, I jumped into the other cage to restrain him. He was mad. We laughed about it years later.

Rico was a boyhood idol of mine. In 1967, he also was the first player to get to Tony Conigliaro when he was beaned by Jack Hamilton's fastball, a pitch that nearly killed Tony C. Rico was the on deck hitter and we spoke about that night many times. Rico so often told me that when Tony C got hit in the head, it sounded like the bat hitting a piece of fruit. That was a very sad night for everyone in Boston.

Years later, after attempting a comeback and suffering several setback, Tony suffered a heart attack in a car his brother Billy was driving through the Callahan Tunnel. After that, Tony was basically like a handicapped person, just living in his house in Swampscott. Rico went to visit him. He said Billy and Sal (Tony and Billy's father) came to the door. They were so happy to see Rico. When Rico walked into the house, he said Tony got up and had a big smile on his face while reaching out to shake Rico's hand. Rico told me Tony's hand grip was like a vise. He couldn't get his hand loose from Tony's. Billy had Tony in pretty good shape, lifting weights, etc. Although Tony could barely speak, he was physically strong. The night Tony got beaned, I remember sitting in my bedroom listening to the game on the radio as we did almost every night. When Tony passed away in 1990, he was only 45 years old.

27.

Dave Caiazzo: The First Inductee Into Malden High's Hall Of Fame

For the first time in Malden High School history, an athletic hall of fame was taking shape. What the local newspaper did was put a ballot in the paper and people could vote for three people out of the long athletic history of MHS. This went on for a few weeks. This was something I would love to be elected into, but from over the many years there were thousands of former players from many sports so I really didn't think I would have a chance. The one thing I had going for me was my success in baseball. Everyone knew me, also.

A few weeks later, I was just coming through the front door of my house. My mother, Angelina, greeted me and said to call Peter Carroll at the high school or go there to see him personally. I figured it might be some good news but I said to myself, "Let's see what he wants." I went to the classroom he was teaching in and he came out. He put his hand out and said, "Congratulations, Dave, you've been selected as one of the five charter members of Malden's Hall of Fame." You couldn't believe how happy I was. The other inductees were John Salmon, Willie Barron, Charlie O'Rourke and Eddie Melanson; quite a group to be inducted with. These were all great selections and, believe me, I was so proud to be in that class. So often I think of it and of all the people who played over so many years. The way they finally selected us was by taking the final ten people with the most votes and then a committee selected five out of the ten. After the selection, someone on the committee asked me how they should do this process in the future. I just told them to do it correctly, not just letting any-one in or they will have major problems. When that happens, someone is always going to say that he or she was better than some person who was inducted. I wanted them to know that to be in a hall of fame is special. As the years went by, I saw that kind of thing happening.

But this night was going to be special. I had to have someone induct me by talking about my accomplishments for a few minutes. The first person who came to mind was Coach V. The more I thought about it after the ban-quet, the more I thought I made a mistake. I should have asked Coach Frank Adorn, my Malden High School coach, to do it. At that time, I was too long away from the high school scene but that would have been the right thing to do. I feel very sorry about that because I am very friendly with Frank. Coach V was more for what I accomplished in college.

Coach V did an outstanding job. He was well-known by everyone around my area by then. They all knew I played for him. When I told coach about my getting into the Hall of Fame and asking him to speak at the time, he had a great line, as he usually does. He said, "Cai, who's going to beat you out for the Hall of Fame around your area, Paul Revere?" He is some-thing special.

We had a tremendous crowd that night. My entire family went, of course. I introduced everyone including my girlfriend, Janet. When I spoke, I talked a lot about my brother Steve. I said he should be up on stage with me. He was an all-around better athlete. I know, as he always said to me, that "no one dominated their sport like you did, Dave," but Steve was a phe-nomenal football player as he was noticed by everyone in the city. He could hit a baseball better than anyone around the city and if you put him on a basketball court, he could compete with anyone. What an athlete! The best I had seen. I realize he's my brother but I have to tell it like it is. I also thanked my Mom, Dad and Joan during that special evening.

When Coach V got up on stage to speak about me, the one thing he said that got everyone's attention was not my accomplishments but what else he said: "Dave Caiazzo is not only one of the great players, he is the greatest kid who ever came to our university." The college has been in existence since 1960. That quote was put in the newspaper.

In the crowd besides family and long-time friends was a man I loved. His name was Ralph Myerow, an older gentleman who I met just a week before the banquet. While at the Malden YMCA one day, I was changing in one of the locker rooms. I heard people talking in the next locker room over. One man said to the other, "Hey, who is this Dave Caiazzo. I read about him in the paper the other day being the first person getting into the Hall of Fame." The article was big in the newspaper. The other person must have known I was nearby and he said, "Quiet, he's in the next room." As I was leaning over to put on my white sneakers, this older, well-dressed man said as he peeked around the locker, "Hi, are you Mr. Dave Caiazzo?" I said, "Yes, I am. Why?" He said, "I just wanted to congratulate you on getting inducted this coming week." I said "Thank you, and who are you?" He said, "My name is Ralph Myerow. I see you around town a lot." I asked him if he liked baseball and he said he loved baseball. "I said, "How would you like to be a guest of mine at the banquet?" He couldn't believe it and said, "Well, that's going to be a big event, are you sure you want me there?" I pulled out a ticket I had in my pocket and said, "Make sure you're there on Friday and be on time."

Ralph was probably about sixty years old at the time but that event made him feel so important and made me feel great that I did that for him. He met everyone in my family for the first time, along with all my friends. That night was the beginning of a long friendship with Ralph that continues to this day. Someone at the Marriott Hotel a few years later said Ralph would probably be dead now if it wasn't for you bringing him out to dinner, meeting people and being so strong a friend to him. He wouldn't hurt anyone. He loved to be around people, especially sports celebrities. I introduced him to Johnny Pesky, Rico Petrocelli, Joe Morgan, Bill Monbouquette, Eric Wedge, Julio Franco, people like that. Steve Bedrosian got a charge out of him, as did Dave Wallace.

My pitching lessons were picking up tremendously by now. I was doing them at Strike-One baseball complex in Burlington which I found out through Rico. The owners were Mark Lombardi and Steve DiStefano. Both were upstanding and quality people. They treated me great. The working relationship was very professional but they also watched me regarding my diabetes. One night in particular stands out. It was a Sunday, usually my busiest day for lessons. I went from 8 a.m. to 7 p.m. straight through. Well, I guess I didn't eat during the day. By the time I was leaving, Steve and Mark were at the desk and noticed I was swaying back and forth. They knew I needed sugar. One of the things with the disease is you get very defensive about it. It's normal. When they said, "Don't go anywhere, we're going to get something at the snack bar to eat." I kept saying, "I'm all right. I'm all right." I knew I wasn't and so did they. I always figured I could make it through the reaction but you just can't. They kept me there as I was denying being in that state but they won out and got me a candy bar. They made me eat it but I think they thought once you eat it, you're fine. Unfortunately, you have to give it more time to get into your system when you are as low as I was.

So I went on my way. I was on the highway heading home. As I was getting off an exit, the police pulled me over. I don't even remember getting to the place where they stopped me. They asked me some questions and I did manage to tell them I was diabetic and I needed more food. They said I was moving from lane to lane on the highway. Next thing I knew, an ambulance came and the emergency people put me on a stretcher and into the ambulance. As the traffic was all backed up, some people driving by recognized me. I was embarrassed but people were yelling out of their cars, "Cai, you all right?"

As I was put inside the ambulance on the stretcher, the emergency person taking care of me asked how I was doing. He said, "I know you're Dave Caiazzo. Aren't you?" I said yes as he put the IV into my arm. He said he was a sports fan and followed me. He was very good at his job. It was nice to see someone who recognizes you and could talk while you're going through that.

I remember I didn't even have anyone at the Melrose-Wakefield Hospital call my family. I just stayed in there for about three hours until they got my blood sugar level to where it was supposed to be. The other problem was getting to my car. It was towed to Stoneham. I had to take a cab to it and then had to pay, of course. What a night! My stubbornness got me in trouble again with the diabetes. I made it again. However, I know it can't last, my luck, that is, doing it my way much longer.

Brother Steve was always harping on me to "slow down," saying I'm doing too much. I need to rest, especially having the diabetes. Russ always would tell me he's never seen anyone do what I do, saying if there was that someone, they'd be dead by now. There was simply no "slow down" in my life. Everyday life was no different than on the baseball field. Just do everything right to the end and don't leave it in anyone else's hands. I didn't want anyone to finish my games nor did I want anyone to pick up where I leave off in everyday life. That wouldn't be Davey Cai.

28.

Scouting For The Cleveland Indians And The Anaheim Angels

SINCE MY DEPARTURE FROM PRO ball, I continued to play semi-pro with the A's. Only now I had to pitch more efficiently but also in severe pain every time out. We were winning championship after championship. Joe D was still player-manager when I was on my second run with the team, and after Joe was John Brickley. They really wanted me to pitch for them again, so I did. Since I wasn't pitching as often as I did in past years, whenever I did pitch, I controlled the game pretty well. Around the year 1980, I pitched in about seven or eight games and I might have lost one close game but won most of them. My earned run average was about 1.00. No one could hit me. Maybe I shouldn't say that but I would strike out my six or seven guys a game, wouldn't give up more than five hits and when they hit me, it was soft stuff, nothing solid.

As we got into the early '80s, my arm was so bad I could hardly sleep, couldn't reach over to open the car window before they had power windows. When needed, one of the coaches or players would call me to pitch. One game in particular was against the Somerville Elms. We were down two games to one in the best-of-five series in the first round of the playoffs. One more loss and we were eliminated. I was at work around 3 p.m. and the telephone rang. It was Freddy Campatelli who was like a player-coach. He said, "Cai, I need a huge favor." I asked what he needed. He said, "You know we have to win tonight. If we win, I know we'll win the series but we need you to get us to that final game. Can you do it?"

"What time is the game?" I asked. He said,"6 p.m." I said, "I'll be there." We won 3-1 and we did win the final game, as well, to go on. Freddy still tells that story to everyone around us when we're together. He made reference that I had balls like this, illustrating with his hands, meaning large.

Right around this period, the Cleveland Indians approached me about scouting in the New England area. The head guy approached me and I met him for the signing. I would cover the high school and college kids in the area. Steve Donaghey was the first kid I had an important part in signing. My boss had asked me to go see a kid in high school from Reading. When I went, I didn't like the kid I was supposed to scout but I did notice Steve D both at the plate and on the mound. He had a presence to him. He was about 6 ft. 5 in. tall and hit from both sides of the plate. He swung pretty good. Then, later in the game with the kid at the plate that I was sent to see, Donaghey was brought in to pitch to him. He blew him away. When I got home, I called my boss and said forget about the kid you wanted me to look at, I found another kid. I wrote the report on him. Later that spring, the Kansas City Royals drafted him in the thirteenth round as an infielder. So, I knew I was on target with this kid.

A few years later, I got a phone call. It was Steve Donaghey. He said, "Dave, I don't know if you remember me." I said, "Of course I do." He said he was at Georgia Tech and just finished a good career but injured his left hand and now was having trouble swinging the bat. He wanted me to work with him and see if I could look at him as a pitcher. I said, "Why not." When I saw him, I said, "Not bad. You're throwing about 86 miles an hour." He said, "That's not good, is it?" I told him he was dragging his back leg which will hamper his velocity but that if we work on that, I thought he could get up to 89 miles an hour. We had three or four lessons and I went to see him pitch in a game. Sure enough, he hit 89 mph.

I immediately called my boss and told him I was going to send him to our final tryout in Poughkeepsie, New York. He said, "No, we've already seen him at the last tryout we had in Lowell." I told him we got his velocity up to 89 mph but my boss said "no" again. Finally I said, "Well, fire me if you like but this kid is going there. I already told him he was going and I'm sending him." I told my boss that I think I've demonstrated that I knew what I was doing and I've given him kids in the past. He finally said "OK."

That day was a Sunday and I had a full schedule of pitching lessons so I couldn't go to the New York tryout but when I got home, I had a message on my phone from Steve D saying he didn't know how to thank me. He had topped off at 91 mph at the tryout and we signed him and I supposedly got credit for the sign. I called my boss and said, "Didn't I tell you?" He said, "You were right."

Steve lasted three years in our system. That was all he wanted, a chance, and I knew he deserved one. Just goes to show you, sometimes the people who think they're the only ones who know, don't.

29.

My Boyhood Idol, Mickey Mantle, Dead

BIG BROTHER STEVE HAD BEEN married to Donna a couple of years now and had a beautiful daughter, Jenna. I was Steve's best man at his wedding. Sister Joan was getting prepared to marry her long-time boyfriend, Jack. My father Rocco was really excited about giving his daughter away. Soon after, Joan and Jack were married and that was a very nice wedding, as well.

Working regularly at the Copley Plaza was exciting and I looked forward to going to work each day. A group of girls from a school in California came to Boston to look at colleges. They were from rich families, from what we heard. They stayed about five nights. Jim Carey and I would often talk to them at the concierge desk. One of the girls I hit it off with was a girl named Kelly. As it turned out, she was a niece of Anheuser Busch. Her mother was his sister. When they were leaving to head to New York to look at schools, they asked us if we wanted to meet them there. Jim and I drove out there a couple of days later and spent a few days in the big city. At the time, my cousin, Nicky Cai, was there doing his modeling and acting so we stayed with him. I remember a few weeks later trying to reach Kelly at one of the four or five houses she gave me phone numbers at. The homes must have been big because each time it was either the butler or someone else trying to track her down, sometimes taking five minutes before she would get to the phone. My cousin Nick met Kelly when we met the girls and he just thought she was special. One of the nights, we went to a nice New York bar and Nick introduced

Jim and I to former NFL running back Ed Marinaro. Kelly and I stayed in touch for quite a while but then we kind of went our own ways. She was a very nice girl and someone would have loved to have her for a trophy some day.

I enjoyed the scouting but was asked to do things that benefitted others but not Dave Cai. I turned my boss onto a kid from New Haven named T.T. Gallagher, an outfielder who could run like a greyhound. When I made the trips to Florida for spring training with New Haven, my boss would ask me to work him out, get his times in the 40-yard dash and 60-yard dash, and his times down the base line. I gave him all the reports. I gave him such great reports that my boss brought Josh Burns down to introduce me to him and personally look at Gallagher. Burns was the director of scouting for the Cleveland Indians at the time but ended up as the general manager of the Arizona Diamondbacks for years. He was, it seemed, a nice guy. As it turned out, we drafted Gallagher that spring. My boss said to me, "Great job, Dave."

Another player I had a hand in signing was a kid from Lexington named Mo Christmas. I got word of him through my now good friend Rico Petrocelli. I notified my boss after I watched him throw for me one day. When my boss worked him and liked him, we signed Christmas, as well. I know I was doing my job well above what a lot of scouts around the area were doing. Not feeling that I was getting much more than a "thanks, Cai," for everything, I was getting a bit annoyed.

We held a tryout camp at the University of Lowell on a weekday. My boss was in charge and there were area people like myself there as well. While working with all the pitchers in the bullpen before they went out to throw live to hitters, I got talking to most every pitcher. My job that day was to evaluate each kid but not to make any corrections in their delivery, etc. This one guy who was a "bird dog" scout for us was telling kids about Rollins College and doing a little recruiting as well for Rollins. His son supposedly was playing ball at Rollins and that is why he was showing a great interest in the college.

He was taking kids' telephone numbers down and it really didn't bother me. As I worked with the pitchers, one in particular I liked. His name was Mike Marini, from Lynn, He threw pretty well. When I asked him where he was committed to college, he said he had a few options but was still unde-cided. I asked him if he had heard of my alma mater, the University of New Haven. He responded, "Of course, that's the best program around." I told him I could help him get in there if he was interested. I told him I was a spe-cial pitching instructor for them during their spring training trip and that I was constantly in touch with their coach, the great Porky Vieira. At the end of the workouts, he said would give me his telephone number, etc. At the end of the workout, he came up to me and thanked me for showing an interest in him and gave me his information.

Apparently my boss saw the exchange and came up to me and said, "David, don't use this as a recruiting session for New Haven." I was fuming! First of all, he was doing a little something at the University of Lowell for the baseball team, which was a rival of New Haven. He didn't think I knew that but being around people all the time, I hear everything. My response to him was simple. "Take your job and I'm out of here. Don't ever tell me I can't help a kid get into school or try to get a family any scholarship money." That was an insult.

You know, these guys who have been involved in baseball only a quarter of their lives think they know everything. My baseball knowledge was from the day I was born. After I started to walk to my car, he came walking after me saying, "Come back. I'm sorry." Sorry wasn't good enough for me. I opened my car door and started to change my shoes and shirt. You knew he knew I wasn't kidding around. I was serious. Dave Caiazzo doesn't embarrass anyone nor should anyone try to embarrass him. He now said that he was treating all the staff at a Bennigan's restaurant or someplace similar and wanted me to come. I said, "I'm not going." He would not leave. After practically begging me to go, I said OK. When we got outside the restaurant, he came up to me again and said he was glad I came. I told him about that other scout recruiting practically on the field and he never said anything to him regarding it. He apologized.

Another local kid from Medford named Justin Crisafulli is someone else I was responsible for signing. I had played against his father Jay for years. Justin was in high school when I first went to see him but turned out to be a good hitter in junior college. I followed him and kept an eye on him in the summer league. Going to see him play five or six games in a row convinced me he deserved a shot. I called my boss to watch him one night and he told me to set up a workout. We did and we signed him to an Indians contract. He didn't play too long but definitely deserved to get a shot.

The highest draft pick I dealt with was a kid I gave pitching lessons to. He came a pretty good distance to see me each Sunday. He lived in Orange, Mass., a good hour and twenty minutes away. His name was Eric Thomas, a big, 6 ft. 9 in. righthander. He came with his dad Mel each week. I saw the progress he was making so I had Coach V look at him for New Haven. He gave him a full ride. In his first year, Eric couldn't break the starting rotation and got a little down on himself. Let's not forget that Coach V was no easy coach to play for. You needed thick skin. After the first year, Eric's dad called me and said he was now thinking of changing to a junior college. I tried to discourage him but he definitely wanted to sign and if you are in junior college, you can after your first year.

Eric had a good year at junior college but then wanted to go to a school down south. They called me and asked my opinion, especially since he did get drafted in the thirteenth round by the Detroit Tigers. What I told Mel was that the offer the Tigers made to Eric wasn't as high as a thirteenth rounder should get and to tell the Tigers they needed more money. Another local kid signed with the Red Sox in the same round and got about $10,000 more. I told them to tell the Tigers that if they don't give him the money, then he'd go on to another four-year school. Mel and Eric called me back and said the Tigers weren't going to give him the money and asked me what to do next. I explained to both of them to trust me and that I would steer them in the right direction. Mel said we trust you more than anyone, that's why we're asking your advice. What I advised was that Eric shouldn't choose a big baseball factory for a school. If he did, he might get lost in the shuffle. He needed to go to a good school where he was going to pitch and get looked at, and I knew he would go a lot higher than the thirteenth round next season and get a ton more money.

They said all right. They decided on a school down south and Eric did well but was hurt after the first five or six games. But the scouts loved him. He was throwing in the mid nineties. Exactly what I said would happen, did happen. The Milwaukee Brewers took him in the third round and gave him a $500,000 bonus. What a score! Mel and Eric couldn't thank me enough. Eric was an intelligent kid who had the arm, as well, to make it. We knew one thing, with that bonus, he was going to be around for a while. Eric lasted about four seasons with the Brewers. Then he called me and said he got released. He had hurt his arm and was rehabbing it. He eventually had the famous Tommy John surgery and got his velocity back up with hard work and rehab.

I called someone to go to Arizona where Eric was now living to take a look at him and, sure enough, we signed him. Only this time it was with my new team, the Anaheim Angels. My boss had switched organizations and asked me to go with him. Eric hung on a couple more seasons before finally calling it a career. But that kid is going to be successful in whatever he decides to do in life. What a super kid he was. He still stays in touch and visits when he's in town. He always says I made an impact on his life.

Right around this time, one of the saddest things in baseball history happened. It was regarding my hero. Mickey Mantle was dying. He had a liver transplant and everyone knew the Mick looked terrible and it wasn't going to be long before his life would be taken away by the abuse of alcohol to his body. Shortly after the transplant, the word around baseball was that he wasn't doing very well. It was getting so bad that the family and Yankees called a number of former Yankee greats who played with Mickey to visit him in the hospital to say their goodbyes. Guys such as Yogi Berra, Whitey Ford, Bobby Richardson, Johnny Blanchard and Hank Bauer all came to the hospital for their final face-to-face with the Mick. A few days later, the Mick was dead.

I was crushed, along with so many millions of baseball fans around the world. Before his death, Mickey had a press conference and said, "This is a role model? Don't be like me." The great Mickey Mantle at sixty-three years old was gone. The man I idolized more than any athlete I've ever seen. All the thrills he gave the baseball world for many years had just passed and we'll never see anyone like him again. I knew I'd be a different person going to a major league game again and not seeing #7 come out of that dugout. What a hero he was to me.

30.

Didn't Have The Strength To Pick Myself Up From The Floor

JOAN WAS MARRIED TO JACK now and Steve's wife Donna was expecting a baby. Everything at this time in my life seemed to be going better than I could ever expect. It was just that damn diabetes. I was having my moments with that. One day I was really scared. I was in my kitchen and I was beginning to cook something to eat because I was getting low. I must have passed out and I found myself on the kitchen floor. It must have been two or three hours before I woke up. When I did, I couldn't pick myself up off the floor. I remember the pan of water I was boiling was evaporated and it was hot, as you can imagine. I was lucky it didn't start a fire, especially while I was unconscious. I couldn't lift myself up off the floor for at least thirty minutes. You see, once you get that low, you can pass out but you eventually wake up. However, it's not good when you do.

Most of the time I wouldn't mention it to anyone, especially anyone in my family. Another time, Kenny Mazonson, a close friend of mine, helped me. Kenny also has diabetes and was one of my long-time instructors at my baseball camp. This day, a mother who was trying to set up a pitching lesson for her son, was trying to reach me by phone. She was trying me for hours and when I didn't answer, she got concerned. She happened to know Kenny and called him to check on me. Kenny lived only a few blocks away so he drove to my condo. When he got there, he found the door unlocked and came upstairs. When he got upstairs, he was amazed. He saw blood everywhere. It looked like there was a murder in the house. What must have happened was I had a glass in my hand when I fell it obviously broke and I cut my hand badly but while trying to get up off the floor, I was touching different things and blood marks were everywhere. An ambulance came and I went to the hospital. Kenny's a good friend. He knows what it is like to go through reactions with diabetes.

I think I happened to tell Steve about this incident. He sat me down and said, "Hey Dave, everyone loves you and we want you around for a while. You have to take better care of yourself and slow down a little."

A short time after that incident, I met a girl through Trixie name Joanie. She did some modeling in Boston. She was a good looker. We would see each other when Trixie would plan something. We would end up finding our way to each other at these times and we ended up going out for different periods of time; nothing steady, but over a few years. She loved sex, and who didn't? She had that look to her that was attractive to any guy that had good eyes. When she dressed up, she had that "wholesome girl" look. One time, I couldn't perform well for her when I was really low. She said "What's wrong?" and started to cry.

The Augustine's A's team was still dominant. We were the most dominant team ever in the Intercity League. The Hosmer Chiefs were on top for a number of years but we soon took that position over with all our championships. Time was getting close for me to think about retiring from baseball altogether. I could only pitch maybe every eight to ten days now. I still wouldn't lose but couldn't do it as often. One night while sitting at home I got a strange call. A woman called me and said she'd been following my career for some time and saved every article and took a lot of pictures. She lived right around the corner from Devir Park where we played. She invited me over to look at her collection. It seemed that she must have been at every game because she had amazing pictures. I forget her name but she was very nice. That was such a nice thing for anyone to do. It was a lot of work.

After so many years at the Copley Plaza hotel and meeting all those great stars and people I worked with, I made a change. I began to work with Fitz-Inn Auto Parks running the garage at the Marriott Long Wharf in Boston. The people were very nice and they ran a great hotel. They had some great general managers when I was there, from John Burgess to Terry Worden to Bill Skoglund to Victor Aragona.

When I was in the garage in my first week, I saw an employee who caught my eye. While entering the cafeteria to eat, I noticed one of the most beautiful women I had ever seen. I asked about her and someone told me her name was Christina and she was a cheerleader for the New England

Patriots. My head couldn't get away from her. She said hello to me one day and we got talking. She worked as the wedding coordinator. She said someone told her I played professional baseball and she asked me to sign a picture for her. I asked her for one of her cheering in return. She said, "That's a deal." A few days later, I gave her my picture and signed it over to her. Then she gave me this huge calendar of all the Patriots cheerleaders. Of all the girls, she was the one they used in a bathing suit picture.

That kind of started things off. She eventually gave me her telephone number. The one thing someone told me about her was she won't go out with anyone. That to me was challenging. I began calling her and we started to go out a lot. The one thing I soon found out was that she was a Mormon. I didn't know too much about that but soon found out. After seeing her quite a bit, she started to let me know that if our relationship got any further, I would have to become a Mormon. For that to happen, I needed to go to her church, etc. She started getting me to go at least once, sometimes twice, a week. I was starting to wonder if my mind was going crazy on me. One day in particular, all the women at the church were cooking for the guys after their church session. Christina was really looking forward to this day. I found out while going to these classes at the church that they were trying to convert me to become a Mormon. I didn't like the feeling I was getting about this but I really loved her. I gave this some serious thought. Then decided when this class was over, I was going right out the back door and heading home. That's exactly what I did; never saw Christina who was cooking in the kitchen with the other girls.

I went home and never picked up the phone. I didn't know how I was going to tell her. Unfortunately for me, we worked in the same hotel. The next day at work, Christina went right to my garage office and was knocking on the door. I couldn't answer it but knew I could not avoid her. Lunch time was coming soon. She was great with everything once we talked and we still went out but we understood it wasn't going to happen. Her last night in Boston after she transferred to California was a very sad night for me. I really, really loved her but seeing her leave after a couple of years was sad. Once she got out to California, she was invited to a big wedding. She called me to invite me to be her guest. I went and we had a great time. After that, though, we just remained great friends, staying in touch.

Steve Ring, my long-time friend who was now living down the Cape, managed a baseball team in the prestigious Cape Cod League (his Harwich team won the playoff title in 1983) before he began coaching in the Cranberry League. Steve had asked me to pitch for him in some of his big games. Coach V had come to visit me in Boston at the same time that Steve called me. When I told Coach V that Steve wanted me to pitch that night down the Cape, Coach said, "Let's go." We jumped in my car and headed down.

I can remember that night like it was yesterday. Steve was telling some of his players "just observe when Dave is out on the mound." I said to myself, "I can't disappoint Stevie." I really didn't know how my arm was going to feel that night but, once again, I knew I was going to win. And Stevie knew that, as well. My arm didn't feel bad but not great either. We scored early and I had a no-hitter going into the ninth inning. It was 2-0 at the time. Everyone knew I had a no-no going. With two outs in the ninth, a kid hit cue shot off his handle just over the second base bag and it just eluded our second baseman's dive. That was the final. After the game, the league's press interviewed me and they also recognized Coach V in the stands. I ended up getting "Pitcher of the Week" honors along with a very nice article on Stevie and me reuniting.

I hadn't thrown in some time so the person more surprised than anyone was Coach V. He came right up to me after the game and said, "Holy Christ. They couldn't touch you. It's like the old days. You can pitch pro ball right now the way you threw tonight." I was just happy to help Stevie out. He ended up wanting me to go down the Cape to pitch more after that game but just a few times was good enough for me. While pitching for Stevie, I never lost. That was fun.

Things back at the hotel garage were going well. Managing most of the guys was fun but you had some who were worse than little kids, always complaining, whining, etc. I let the guys be guys but work had to be done. Even though I worked for Fitz-Inn, I was there representing the Marriott Long Wharf. One slow day, the guys were trying to knock a cup off a trash can from about sixty feet away. It seemed that they were trying for an awfully long time. Finally I said, "You guys are still trying to knock that cup off? Give me the ball and we'll end this." I grabbed the tennis ball and on the first throw, I knocked it off, hitting it square. The guys were amazed. I said, "Let's get to work now. You guys would have been here for a couple of days." I couldn't disappoint.

The hotel was organizing an event for the employees to attend. It was called something like "We Do It Better." The marketing director and GM asked me if I could get a person in the sports field to speak at the time. I made my calls and got Kevin McHale and Robert Parrish of the Celtics to come. People at the Marriott were thrilled and both McHale and Parrish did an outstanding job. My friend Eddie Rideout was really responsible for helping me get those two greats.

I tried to treat the guys in the garage like men; I realized they will respect you more. I never asked anyone to respect me. That's not something you have to ask for; you earn it by your actions. Habib Rehman in the garage was someone who I respected. He was a little older but was in tip top shape for someone his age. He would always tell me to send my mother in to say hello to him at his second job at Downtown Crossing in Boston. My Mom would go shopping there but never stop in to see Habib because he wanted to give her gift certificates, and she felt funny about receiving them. Habib was such a nice man, very respectful. He gave me a bunch of certificates so finally I talked my Mom into going in for lunch. Once she went in, she loved it and Habib made her so comfortable, she went back. He was really nice to her. Men like Habib made the job worth it.

Pierre was another outstanding person in the garage; just a nice, down-to-earth, hardworking guy that I had a lot of respect for. Jamie Palacio, who works in the concierge lounge, is another great guy. He always calls me his "living legend."

When brother Steve and Donna had their baby, Jenna, what a beautiful child! They asked me to be the godfather. I remember Rocco walking around the house really slow, holding her in his arms trying to get her to sleep and just talking extremely softly to her. She was only a few months old at the time.

Being asked to speak at banquets was getting to be a regular thing. I spoke at about six of seven baseball banquets and at the Kiwanis Club of Malden, as well. There were so many more. It was fun doing those. The city of Everett asked me to do a baseball clinic for their entire baseball program. That went very well. I had a few of the instructors from my camp join me to help and instruct. The city of Malden also asked and did a great clinic at Ferryway Green park.

The summer camps were going great, continually growing each year. It seemed each year I would end up taking out a mother of one of the kids; single moms that is. Every year a mother would come to meet me when signing up her son at the park on the first day. When they would call me over, my instructors such as Ernie Ardolino, Chris Nance, Johnny Brickley and John Carco would say, "Look at this one waiting to meet Dave." "That's a definite comp," they would add, kidding around. One mother was a Malden police officer named Carole. She had a nice boy named Michael. We ended up going out for a while, nothing steady but it was a fun relationship. She was and still is a wonderful girl and a terrific mother to Michael. The guys at the camp would get wound up when she would come into the park each morning. They would tease me by saying, "We don't know how you can afford to pay us when all these good-looking mothers get comped." That wasn't true, however.

A friend of mine, Tommy Barros' wife, one day told me she worked with Robin Bavaro. Robin was the sister of the New York Giant great tight end Mark Bavaro and his brother David Bavaro. Also, her father was my old history teacher Tony Bavaro at Beebe Junior High. What a small world. She wanted us to get together. We met and we went out a number of times. She was a wholesome-looking woman. She was very attractive. She held some big jobs with the MBTA, the Corrections Dept., and later worked for House Speaker Tom Finneran.

A short time later, my old high school coach Frank Adorn called me and asked if I was interested in working Mark Bavaro's camp. I would be doing the pitching part of it with the kids. I did that for about five years. Mark was a great guy. He definitely got a bad rap from the media about his personality. He was just a very quiet, soft spoken guy. I can't say enough about him and his dad Tony. Dick Beredino, the long-time baseball coach with the Red Sox, was one of the instructors. He knew Tony because they went to Holy Cross together. When he was coaching at Lowell for the Red Sox farm club, I stopped by to say hello. When I went to the dugout before the game, I asked someone if Dick was available. He said, "I don't think so. He won't come out." I told the person "just tell him it's Dave Caiazzo." Not more than fifteen seconds later, out came Dick with that big smile. What a wonderful human being and what a book of baseball information he has stored in that head of his.

Besides the summer camp, I extended a private pitching clinic for no more than twenty kids. John Carco and I conducted it. John and I were teammates on Augustine's for a couple of summers. I used to tease John by saying, "I do all the work and you make a nice piece of change." He and I really hit it off. He used to throw batting practice for the Red Sox. John threw pretty hard. But I'd say to John, "I would have hated to be Wade Boggs or Jim Rice hitting against you, trying to get their strokes down with a pitch coming at their head." John had a bit of wildness at times but knew how to pitch. We did this for about five or six years. He also worked and coordinated my camp for a few years.

I was seriously thinking of ending my pitching days. It was pretty definite. This was going to be my last season. My arm couldn't take it any more. My last year was one in which I pitched occasionally. Andy Brickley, John Brickley and our beloved Harry Mehos were just amazed at how I got by with the pain I was enduring and with the velocity I was throwing at. I had to locate. Staying ahead with not just first pitch fastball was the key.

Command is the pitcher's biggest asset. If you have command of two or three pitches, you can start hitters off with changeups, curves, sliders, whatever, and you'll be so much more effective. Not every batter should get a first pitch fastball. That's what I was now doing; that's why I continued to win.

In my last season, I pitched a game against Wilmington. The umpire was a man I'd seen behind the dish for years. His last name was Tighe. During that game I had no velocity but I spotted everything well and used all my pitches. I had a no-hitter into the fifth inning and we had a small lead. When I threw a pitch in the sixth inning, someone hit a line drive back at me. I couldn't react fast enough, like the old days, and it hit off my finger that I had sticking out of my glove. I broke the finger but no one knew. I stayed in the game but gave up two hits and we won. Was that finger sore! All my years I never got hit with a ball batted back to me.

After the game, the umpire Tighe made his way over to me and said, "Dave, that was unbelievable. I saw how much pain you were in out there and that was a treat to be able to umpire your game." That was nice of him to make it over to me and say that. He knew that was maybe my last start. It wasn't. I had one more and did well but the big thing was that we won another championship and it was the end for most of the guys on the A's, as well. Some did continue to play.

31.

New Haven Hall Of Fame, But Rocco Couldn't Be There

MOM AND DAD WOULD MAKE a yearly trip to Poland Springs, Maine. They loved it there but this year was going to be the last. We got the biggest scare while sitting at home relaxing. Rocco wasn't well. You knew he wasn't by the look on his face. I went into the living room to check on him. He was barely breathing. Mom and I called an ambulance. In the meantime, I called Steve and told him to come right over. When the ambulance came, they administered to Dad for a few minutes as we all watched. Joan was in Methuen so she couldn't get to the house by the time the ambulance arrived. Steve, Mom and I were in shock. My heart was in my mouth. I was just praying Dad would make it. Mom was confused. She didn't know what to do. The driver said they were bringing Dad to Malden Hospital. We got Mom squared away and made our way to the hospital. He was doing better after a few hours went by. We stayed there for hours but they said he was doing better and we could go home. They were keeping Dad on a monitor.

We were there every day to visit him constantly. By now he was in there three days and he was speaking very well and was in good spirits. After the third night, I believe I was the last one of us to see him that evening. I had worked and Mom, Steve and Joan were visiting him earlier in the day. I went to visit directly from work. I stayed at Mom's that night and about 4 a.m. the telephone rang. I woke up but Mom answered it. I had a bad feeling. Who would call at that hour? I made my way to listen outside Mom's room and heard her crying and talking. I knew something with Dad had happened and it wasn't anything good. When Mom hung up, I opened the door and said, "What happened, Mom?" She said that was the hospital and Dad took a massive heart attack and they couldn't revive him. When I heard that, it was the loneliest day of my life. But I had to stay strong for Mom. We called Steve and Joan to tell them. With Joan, we had to tell Jack to tell her since he answered the phone and Joan can get very emotional about Dad.

We planned the funeral with help from Uncle Cliff. He did a tremendous job helping us. We had so many important people to call to send their condolences. One call in particular was to Cy Young Award-winner Steve Bedrosian. He loved my Dad. The funeral was huge. People said one of the largest they had seen. That made us all feel good because I believe if you were a good person in life, it will be noticed at your funeral. Coach Vieira made a special trip for the funeral. Coach respected Rocco as much as anyone. Coming from Coach V. that's a tremendous compliment. He didn't give out compliments very often. He used to say, "You're father's a peach."

Trying to prepare for the final day was going to be awfully difficult. We had so much support from everyone that it made everything much easier. We were all so close with Dad but Joan, I think, took it the hardest. We all cried endlessly but seeing Steve break down showed us all how much he loved his father especially when we made our final visit to the open casket. That was difficult. Not seeing our father any longer was something we couldn't prepare for. After just a few days, I already missed him dearly. People would come to give us their condolences in line at the funeral parlor and people would comment how, even in the casket, he looked so handsome. It marked the end of a great era.

Life had to go on. Joan and Jack had Bethann not long after and Melissa followed a few years later. I was again another godfather, this time to Bethann.

Shortly after Dad passed, I got a great letter in the mail from the University of New Haven. The written part of the letter said, "Cai, congratulations, you are now a member of the Charger Hall of Fame." It was written by Coach V. What news! There were only three or four baseball players chosen before me. The history of our program showed how difficult it was to get inducted after all the great players we've had there. So I was humbled, to say the least. Coach Vieira was going to introduce me at the event. The Athletic Department sports information director must have contacted everyone. The local newspaper did a big spread on it and then the Boston Herald sports department called. Rich Thompson, the long-time writer, called me and wanted to do an interview. He came to the Marriott Long Wharf and interviewed me for about a half an hour.

A week or so later, I began getting calls from everywhere saying they got the Sunday paper and there was a huge article on me. It was part of the regular weekly section titled "Whatever Happened To." It was done each week on people who had illustrious careers but then kind of fell out of touch with a lot of people. The first thing I did was get a couple of copies. The article covered the entire page. I got one for the house and the other to put on Rocco's grave. In the article, it mentioned how he had just passed not long before this and how inspirational he was in my life and baseball career. The article stated how I "did everything to please him." I signed a copy and put it on his grave. I wrote, "Dad, this one's for you."

The next big event in my life was coming up – the Hall of Fame banquet. We had three car loads of people go, including my family members and friends. A girl I was seeing at the time also came. Her name was Donna. She was from Medford. I had to get to the hall early for pictures and interviews.

I was pleased so much to be inducted along with my college catcher Pat Murphy. He was something. When you talk about steady ballplayers, he comes to mind right away. Not only that, but he's also a great kid. The other person being inducted was Miles McPherson, a football player. That year his brother at Syracuse, Don McPherson, was a Heisman Trophy candidate and finished as the runnerup to Tim Brown.

No one could have asked for a better introduction than the one Coach V gave me. He spoke for ten minutes. The thing that stood out more than anything was when he said, "Dave performed at a level you just can't believe." Coming from him, I had tears in my eyes. The other thing that stood out was when he said, "Never mind talking about being tough. Cai was the toughest I've seen between the white lines."

The plaque read: "The only thing harder than scoring runs off Dave Caiazzo was beating the righthander. Caiazzo registered six career shutouts, the second-best total in UNH history, and won 22 of 24 decisions. These numbers become more impressive when you consider Caiazzo accomplished this in only two years. His only losses were 1-0 and pitching on one day's rest."

As far as I was concerned, my baseball career was complete. For all I worked for, I was rewarded. Some of the people you had to deal with along the way made it more difficult but I made it through. Nothing's more difficult than facing a family death and dealing with that. I thought having the bases loaded with no one out and a three-ball, no-strike count on the batter in the bottom of the ninth inning was tough. Not so. That was a cake walk for me compared to Dad's death. Habib used to say to me, "Dave, remember you only have one mother and one father. You have to take care of them as long as you can." Boy, was he right!

There was a real jerk who kind of made me choose not to stay in the restaurant bar business any longer. When I was filling in at the bar at my Pub one day until the bartender showed up, a guy came to the bar and ordered a Budweiser beer. I got it and placed it down on the bar in front of him. A few minutes later he said to me, "Is Dave Caiazzo here?" I said, "That's me. Why?" Next thing he did was proceed to ask me personal questions about being in baseball and about the number of women I must have slept with. At that point, I handed him back his money and told him to drink up and leave. Those are the kinds of people who make life bad for everyone.

Jealousy is the worst emotion someone can have. It's the toughest thing to live with. I was never jealous of anyone and never had a reason to be. But I couldn't imagine saying I wish I was like this person. You have to make yourself better than that person so you don't need to think like that.

I've always been a person who got along with the good people but also most of the bad people I may have come in contact with. But most bad people have those skeletons that are coming out. I'm not saying that everyone who may not be a classy individual can turn it around but at least, try.

The mannerisms of some people really bothered me. If they acted like an idiot, then there's no two ways about it, they're an idiot. The way someone is brought up usually is reflected in that person. I know over the years I've been an outspoken person but it was always regarding the way I was going to perform. I wasn't shooting my mouth off about something I had no clue about. If I was hitting or pitching against a team or person and someone asked me what I thought the outcome would be, I'd just tell them. The only person who gets hurt in a situation like that is me if I don't back it up. Russell, growing up, always said to people, "No matter what Dave says, you know he's going to back it up. That's Davey Cai."

The game of baseball was definitely changing. These aluminum bats were really starting to bother me. At the time I was in college, the metal bats came out but then after a number of years, they lowered the sizes. I picked up one and said, "Who the heck can't hit with one of these bats?" Rico Petrocelli and I used to talk about it all the time. I mentioned to him one day that if you're a .280 hitter with the metal then really you're about a .190 hitter. That's how much of a difference it makes.

One day Rico and I were going to lunch. He came by my house on Estey Street to pick me up. I brought him down my cellar and said "pick this aluminum bat up." He said Wow! What's this?" I told him that was the bat I swung when metal first came out. It was so heavy you could barely lift it. So these kids today think they're so great if they're hitting .290 or even .300. Give us a break! Rico and I often talked about how when he was playing, you generally got one pitch per at bat to hit and if you didn't hit it, you weren't getting another one. Today, these hitters are getting two, three and sometimes four pitches per at bat. The pitching is that bad today.

Now that I wasn't playing any baseball anymore, I was going out to listen to good music at clubs. One night a bunch of us went to a place in Middleton run by Richie Conigliaro, Tony's brother. It was called Legends. As I was sitting down talking to some friends I ran into, I spotted this beautiful brunette. I could see she was starting to leave with some other girls she was with. I stopped her and asked where she was going. She said she had a wedding to go to the next day and had to get home. We talked for a few minutes, then she gave me her telephone number at a hotel where she was staying. She was from Alaska and worked for Alaska Airlines. One of my buddies I was with called her a "showpiece." Jenny was her name. She was something to look at. The next day I called her and she told me she was leaving the next morning after the wedding. She had a great job. She was in charge of security at the airport in Alaska.

We stayed in contact and she was single. How lucky could I be! A few months later I made my plans to go to California as I usually do in the fall. We made plans to meet in Newport Beach. She flew for free because she worked for the airline. I made arrangements when she came in to have a separate room for her and me because Ralph Myerow joined me for the trip to California. Ralph gave me my time with her alone, although she could only stay two nights because she had to be back at work. We had an exciting two days. She dressed just the way I liked women to dress, classy and casual. She looked outstanding in her jeans and we just meshed. We had dinner one night at an exceptional Italian restaurant. Slept in the next morning and went for a great brunch. I don't think either of us wanted to leave each other. The time went by pretty quickly. Ralphy still had a good eye for the women and thought Jenny was a knockout. She left two days later and I really thought we could end up together.

But, once again, my schedule combined with hers didn't allow that to happen. We stayed in contact and she kept asking me when we were going to see each other again. I think she thought I kept putting her off and she was getting upset. She kept asking why such a handsome guy wasn't married. I kept telling her that what girl would want to take care of a guy who had diabetes. She knew I was joking about that. After a number of months, she was really getting annoyed. I could tell in her voice, obviously, because I couldn't tell by her facial expressions. After another month or so, we ended it. Too bad, because she was a top notch girl.

Steve's daughter Jenna and Joan's two daughters Bethann and Melissa were starting to grow up. Mom was doing all right for someone who lost her husband but she was staying in a lot. As much as we tried getting her out of the house, she stayed in and watched television in the living room. Friends of mine such as Phil D'Amore would stop by Mom's house to say hello to her and comment how great she looked. She was in her seventies but looked to be sixty, at the most. She did look outstanding.

The baseball lessons were going very well. Mark Lombardi and Eric Wedge had a fundraiser at the Dennisport Yacht Club. They were having celebrities such as former Red Sox manager Joe Morgan and former Red Sox pitcher Bill Monbouquette, along with many others. When I arrived, I was looking for Bill Monbo and saw him talking to Joe Morgan. I walked over to them and put my arm around Bill and said, "It's been years but you used to scout me for the Yankees and gave me a great recommendation for college. Do you remember me?" He thought for a second, then smiled and said, "Yeah. Joe Pepitone." I laughed and said, "No, he's my cousin. I'm Dave Caiazzo." He remembered. Joe Morgan was very friendly that night, also.

Mac Singleton, my old gym teacher at Beebe Junior High, called me one day. He said, "Are you interested in coaching any more?" He knew I had helped Bobby Ware at Malden High years ago and knew about coaching at New Haven and the scouting, as well. He was coaching at MIT and wanted me to throw to his hitters during batting practice and then get me in as the pitching coach. I went down and threw BP to his team at Tufts before their game. He said it was the best BP he'd ever seen. He said I must have thrown about 100 pitches and maybe threw one ball. I did it again at MIT and Mac was very happy with me. He kept giving me some good money to do it. At first, I didn't want to take it but he said he was budgeted for it. Then he sent me a contract to be the pitching coach.

Mac was an outstanding athlete in his day and a great individual. He was in the Malden High Hall of Fame. He had been the head football coach at Boston State College. He also was a pro with the Green Bay Packers and the Boston Patriots. He always showed a great interest in me growing up so I really liked Mac and I decided to take the pitching coach position. I wanted him to succeed.

When I joined the MIT coaching staff, I didn't know what to think. I was used to the University of New Haven with all great ball players. These kids just seemed like know-it-alls with not much talent. As much as we worked with them, they couldn't adjust. We had one pitcher I know I helped. He was a Texas boy, Jason Szuminski. He could throw and he listened pretty much; didn't have all the answers like a lot of the players. He went in the tenth round to the Chicago Cubs and made it for a cup of coffee to the majors.

When I look back, I remember one incident that stands out. We were playing at MIT and our starter was tiring so I went to the mound to talk to him. When I got back to the dugout, I told a kid to warm up quickly. As the starter was laboring, I said he's not going to make it past one or two more hitters. He walked the next batter. I looked down to the bullpen and didn't see anyone warming up. I walked toward the dugout and said, "Where's Roscoe?" the pitcher who was supposed to be in the pen. The guys said he went in the direction of the lockerroom. That was about 300 yards behind the field. I looked down and saw him walking toward the school. I yelled, "Roscoe, where are you going?" He yelled back that it was too cold and he needed to warm up inside the gym. I said, "Are you kidding? When do you think I need you, next week?" That's what I'm talking about with these kids. Boy, was it frustrating!

In another game, against Springfield College, my pitcher had a 2-1 lead in the last inning. He got the first two outs and was one out away from a victory but gave up two hits. I took a trip to the mound and explained to him not to give this next batter anything good to hit. I said let's work off the plate and see if he helps by going fishing a little. I barely made it back to the dugout when I heard the sound of contact of wood on the baseball. I looked and it was a base hit to center field scoring both runners and they won the game. What a stupid mistake! Never did what I wanted. Those kids were so smart, they're stupid, sometimes. That's what Mac had to deal with.

A few years later when Mac Singleton asked me to hook on with him at MIT, a funny incident happened. We left Boston and had a connecting flight from Pittsburgh to California. When we arrived in Pittsburgh, we had an hour before catching our next flight out. Assistant head coach Doug Linehan and I said let's ask Mac if he wants to go for a quick cup of coffee. We asked him but he said he was just going to read and he'd be by the gate. Doug and I started to look for a sports memorabilia store I remembered seeing at the airport the last time I was there. We went looking and then kind of lost track of time but still got back to the gate about twenty-five minutes before the flight was leaving. When we got to the gate, we didn't see one person sitting around. We looked at each other and walked up to the gate where there was an airline official. We handed him our tickets and he said, "Sorry, you missed the flight. Everyone has already boarded. We said, "Well, open the door, the flight's not for another twenty-five minutes." The man said, "Sorry, we close the door after everyone has boarded the plane and we don't reopen them." Doug went crazy. He said we got the MIT base-ball team on that flight and we have to drive the vans from the airport to the hotel and we have to be there. He didn't budge. At one point, the official called over his supervisor to help him with Doug and I. The supervisor said that the plane was in the air and Doug responded, "Well, get it down." I almost started to laugh but it was no laughing matter. They told us the next flight to Los Angeles would be two hours after the team would land. We had to come up with another plan. We finally said that we could catch a plane that would take us to Ontario, California. But that was the only way for us to head the team off at the pass. But once we got there we had to take a lim-ousine to our hotel to try to get there before they did. We didn't know who was going to drive those vans. Doug and I split the cost but it was about two hours away from the hotel so we had a long ride.

We said, "Mac's going to kill us when we get there." We finally made it and they beat us by only about thirty minutes. We gave the driver a pretty good tip and jumped out at the hotel. We got to Mac's room and he was laughing. He said, "What happened to you guys?" He said a couple of the players were saying Coach Cai and Coach Linehan never made the flight and they were asking where we were. It was the only flight I have ever missed. Honestly. But we got some laughs out of that one. Mac was saying one of the captains was teasing saying those two guys must have run into a couple of girls at the airport. They always had all the answers. Doug and I killed them on the field when we got there. Doug was a former professional catcher for the New York Mets and also played professional football for the Washington Redskins under Vince Lombardi. He also caught knuckleballer Wilbur Wood in high school. A great athlete. We got along great during out time at MIT. Doug and I got along so well he kept telling me he wanted to set me up with his sister-in-law. When we went to California, that's where she lived. She came to the games and that's where I met her. She would come to Boston to visit her sister and we would go to dinner or meet up at Doug's place in York Beach, Maine. Nothing serious, though. I loved being around Mac and Doug but really found it to be straining to try to coach those kids at MIT who really didn't want to be taught. They all had the answers but none of the answers were right. Just a shame because Mac, Doug and I put all our efforts into coaching them but we got no satisfaction out of it. Doug would coach first base. I used to watch his response con-stantly when kids were running down to first. He was so disgusted that kids weren't running hard down the line or not running through the bag. He would turn his head once they got pretty well up the line. It got so bad at one point that they wanted to make out the lineup card. Mac, of course, always did that. One time when they were saying they didn't agree with the lineup before the game, Doug told them to shut up and knock off the bullshit. He really disliked those kids. Very few of them were going anywhere special in baseball. At the most, they'd be playing softball in the near future but not the real game of baseball.

We coached there for a few years and then we had had it. Mac had a disagreement with the athletic director and ended up getting fired but, believe me, he did not deserve to be. But it was better for him with all the aggravation he went through; taking out of his own pocket to buy kids lunch, etc. He shouldn't have had to do that. But he was that type of person, very giving and generous.

Right around the time Mac and all the coaches left MIT, the E Club of Everett called me. They wanted to honor me at Spinelli's function room on Route One in Peabody for a performance against Everett High School. They did this every year, honor an opposing player who had a great performance. They remembered the game I struck out twenty batters in just eight innings. Larry Vozzella, the head of the E Club, called and said the others at the head table with me would be former Everett great Pat Hughes of the New York Giants, Joe Fitzgerald, the great Boston sportswriter, and Rick Middleton of the Boston Bruins. Everyone was at this banquet; big crowd. Mac Singleton, Doug Linehan (who I coached with at MIT), and about 300 other people were in the audience.

At the end of the event, Rick Middleton came up to me and said, "Dave I have to admit that was as good a speech as I've ever heard." I loved speaking at banquets and events. That made me feel good. At one point in my speech I mentioned my distant relative who played at Everett High years ago. His name was George Caiazzo. People for years had told me he was the greatest football player ever out of that school. Mac also told me that many times. As soon as I mentioned his name, the crowd stood up and cheered. People were aware that he had died just a few months before.

A lot of the newspapers were talking about Johnny Pesky. They said he was losing a lot of weight and was in the hospital not knowing what the problem was. The first thing that came to mind was, at his age, maybe this is the end for him. It sounded as if he was dying. After months, I finally saw where he had been diagnosed as being allergic to flour and now his doctors were trying to get it under control. Johnny was a great guy and I was so happy that the problem wasn't cancer. Rico and I used to talk about his problem.

Just a few months later, I was not feeling well at all; losing weight and feeling like I had no energy. I was practically living in the bathroom; couldn't explain to anyone what was happening. People everywhere were asking me, "Dave, you're losing weight?" I'd always say no but I definitely was and I knew it. I was now working at the concierge department at the Marriott. I would have diabetic reactions there sometimes three or four times a day. I really thought I was going to die; could not explain it to anyone. I'm not a guy who goes to doctors, so I wasn't doing that. Sometimes I would be working and I didn't know where I was. People said I'd be staring and not responding. I didn't even want to go to work each day. I wouldn't even go out of the house much. I wasn't seeing much of my family so they couldn't tell how I was.

One day after work, I was walking to the subway to get to my car. I must have been so low with my blood sugar that I was walking around Boston for three or four hours, not knowing where I was. Somehow I found a subway but was nervous that I might fall into the pit where the tracks are. Two people asked me if I was all right. Of course, as usual, I just said yes; never looking for any help or assistance. When I finally made it to my car at the train station in Malden, I could not find my way home and ended up in Wakefield somewhere. Somehow, I did make it home and collapsed on the couch. I managed to get myself up and eat something. This was happening each day. Even the girls I worked with would get nervous. They would call security to check on me. I think everyone was scared to ask me how I was because, as I said earlier, I would get very defensive due to the severity of my condition. Maria Moreno, the sweetest girl in the hotel and a very good friend of mine, was very concerned about my health.

I kept losing more weight and finally said "enough!" I called and made an appointment at the Joslin Clinic in Boston. When I got there, they said I needed to take four shots of insulin a day now. I was really upset about that. I had taken only one shot a day for more than thirty-five years. But I said I have to do what's best for me. I did this for about a week and called the Joslin back and told them I felt worse than I had before I saw them. I kept eating a lot of bread and pasta to see if I could regain some of my weight. The Joslin said to just keep taking the four daily shots of insulin. I knew there was something really wrong so I suggested to them that I take a blood test. They had me come in and they took the test. They said I would get a call back from them in a day or two. Sure enough, the doctor called me back. I was told I had celiac disease. I said, "What's that?" It's the same thing Johnny Pesky has, exactly. The only thing that may have been good from this was maybe I could go back to one shot a day of insulin. When I went in to meet with the doctor, he said I still had to stay with the four shots.

This was terrible. I found out the reason I was having all the major reactions while at home and work was due to the intake of wheat products I couldn't handle; so everything inside my body was not being kept inside me. This was causing me to have no food in my system with the insulin I was taking and making my blood sugar extremely low. The hotel was extremely attentive to my situation and did not give me any problems with what I was dealing with. I certainly didn't know what was causing this at the time.

A short time after they detected this, Johnny Pesky called and said he heard what I had was the same as his disease. He told me where to shop for my food and what was good to cook and where to get other things such as pastries that were gluten-free, etc. He was great. Once again, I consider myself very lucky to have the amount of friends I have and the quality of friends, as well. If you treat people well, they will treat you well. After at least a year, I was starting to feel normal again. The celiac is no joke. You can die from it very easily without proper care. Wheat is in just about everything. I couldn't even lick a postage stamp. There is wheat in that.

I came in contact with another sister of a professional ballplayer. A friend of mine from Medford, John Aquino, who was a great athlete from that city, was being inducted into the Mustang Hall of Fame. John invited me to go. Charlie Pagliarulo, father of former Yankee third baseman Mike, was being inducted, as well. Charlie was one of my instructors a year or two at my summer camp; just a great person, and family, as well. While at the banquet, sitting at one of the tables, I couldn't help but notice a striking woman. I couldn't keep my eyes off her. I asked Johnny Aquino who she might be and he said he thought she was Mike's sister. I made a few calls after that evening to get any information on her that I could. They said she wasn't married but was seeing some guy from Medford. Word got back to her somehow and she checked out the pictures from that evening and sorted me out at the table.

Somehow I got her telephone number and decided to call her. I knew we wouldn't be without good conversation because of her mom and dad, who I got to know, and Mike, who played on the World Champion Minnesota Twins team in 1991 with my friend Steve Bedrosian. Her name was Lisa. She said she had been down to my Pub in years past. She was going on and off with her boyfriend. I don't think anyone in the family was happy with that situation. We would talk on the phone quite a bit as time went on; easy person to talk to and a magnificent-looking dark-haired beauty. She finally agreed to meet me. We decided to go for a nice dinner and talk. When I was driving to pick her up I was very nervous. I still get nervous with any attractive girl. That's good. If you're not nervous, most likely you don't have feelings. Similar to pitching, people would ask me before a game "Are you nervous?" Of course I am, because I care.

When I got to the house she was as beautiful as I could have imagined. She went into her room to pick up her coat and purse. When she came out she said to me, "You know who you remind me of?" I couldn't bear to hear who she was going to say. She said, "David Hasselhoff," the star of Bay Watch. That was a compliment. She said every time she watched the show she would think of me. That definitely was a plus. However, I didn't want to be compared with anyone. I just wanted to be me. An old friend of mine a few years back used to tell me I reminded him of Baltimore Orioles righthander Jim Palmer. But as great as he was on the mound and as good looking as he was, I used to say I'd rather just be Dave Caiazzo.

That night went great with Lisa, and we said we would get together soon. I didn't want to interfere with her current boyfriend even thought it seemed they were having problems. The best day we had together was when she called me and asked me to pick her up and asked if we could go away for the day. I picked her up and we drove to York Beach, Maine. We walked around, talked and had a great lunch. I could see she was a sweetheart of a girl. She was starting to have big problems with the boyfriend and she wanted to explain it to me. Her mother, Mrs. Pags, would always say that I saved her by getting her away that day. She said, "I'll never forget what you did for Lisa that day." I really don't know what happened but I think it had something to do with her seeing her ex again and I kind of lost touch with her. "Another one by the boards" as people would tease me on. I would hear this on meeting different people and dating.

32.

"Dave, You're The Greatest Pitcher Who Didn't Make It All The Way To The Major Leagues

AN OLD PITCHING COACH I had about the time I was in Legion ball saw me on the street one day. Steve called to me, "Davey Cai." I stopped and it took me a while to realize who he was. I hadn't seen him in about ten or twelve years. He is one nice guy. He asked what I was doing these days and brought up a lot of things I couldn't even remember that happened between the lines. That was good conversation. When we parted, I remember he said, "You were the greatest pitcher that didn't make it all the way to the major leagues. You still look like you can pitch."

There were a couple of kids locally who were doing pretty well now. Richie Barker, one of my private students and former campers, was with the Chicago Cubs. Kevin McGlinchey, also a former camper, was with the Atlanta Braves. Kevin asked me years later to help him with his mechanics and try to help him get hooked on to another organization. Both of these kids were very respectful to me. As always, I tried to help some of the local kids as best I could.

Clean living was what I always thrived on. Take all of those drugs and alcohol and stay clear of me. Russ always said to people that I lived a very clean life with nothing in my system that would make me make a fool of myself. When people would ask me why I didn't drink, I would tell them I don't drink so I can watch some of the comedy that goes around the people who do.

The scouting was still OK. I recommended a kid from my alma mater who was looking to sign. He had a pretty good arm. Coach V asked if I could help him get a contract with us. His name was Ed Sempe. He wasn't a big kid but threw with pretty good arm action. I had him work out for my boss, who liked him and signed him. He lasted about a year and a half or so before getting released. A scout who I liked a lot was a guy named Dave Soper from Saugus. He and I stayed in touch pretty often. He had a pretty good sense of baseball. Any time I would go blank on a kid's name and asked Dave, he would remember it. Dave and I hit it off pretty good. He would ask me things about kids I may have seen and vice versa. Bob Ware, who I coached with at Malden High (he was the head coach then) did some scouting with the Kansas City Royals. We got along great. A real baseball lover; always asking me things about baseball, especially pitching, so that he could improve his knowledge. He had a good baseball head; always enjoyed talking with Bob. He was a little before my time but from what people tell me, he was a pretty good pitcher in his day. He was from Chelsea. He had a nice family and always said to me, "I wish I knew you when my son Bobby was born. I would have made you his godfather." Nice compliment that was. Bob's still doing well and always stays in touch with me. Bob's one of those people you don't mind running into pretty often.

Another knowledgeable baseball guy I became very friendly with was a close friend of Coach V. His name is Tony Asman. I call him Tony O. He's a great man who loves the game of baseball. When Coach V would have me make the annual trip to Daytona Beach, Florida, to work with his college pitchers, Tony would make the trip, as well. Tony grew up with Coach V and used to play against him in sports. Tony O was a Providence College grad who pitched there.

I'll never forget one day down south we were playing a game (New Haven against Tiffin College). At the baseball complex, it is set up where there are three or four fields surrounding each other. This particular day Tony was watching our game behind third base when a foul ball from one of the other fields came in his direction. Tony picked it up and some of us were looking because people were yelling to watch out for the ball being hit. There was an older man heading toward Tony to retrieve the ball from him in order to give it back to the game where the ball came from. The man may have been eighty or so years old. He was waving his hands for Tony either to underhand it back or roll it to him. For some reason, Tony still has that competitiveness in him and he wound up like he was pitching and threw what seemed like a fastball at the man and hit him on the forehead. The man went down like a ton of bricks. Tony imitates the look on my face when he hit the guy. I was shocked. Tony ran over to him and said, "I shouldn't have thrown the ball back to him in the first place." Tony, Coach V and I never laugh on any subject like we do with that story after I imitate how Tony wound up and threw a pill at the old timer. They got the man up eventually and he was OK but Tony made that day memorable. Some twenty years later we laugh to no end on that story. Tony is a funny guy.

Settling in as a confirmed bachelor was something I really didn't want to do. As much as I went out at night and dated so often, I didn't want people to say "Dave's just a bachelor, never got married." I wanted to be married, believe me. I was always very cautious of who I was with and didn't want to take a chance on someone I wasn't quite sure of. Even the girls who seemed right for me, I just seemed to drift away from. Mom would always say, "David, oh you have to meet a nice girl and get married. Mom was always looking out for us kids, as did Dad when he was around. Steve separated by now from Donna and was living with Susan Cicciarelli. She was a Malden girl. They seem to be a fixture. They are not married, though. She adores Steve and I know the feeling is mutual with him. Not too long ago I teased Steve when I was visiting him. I said, "Are you sure you didn't get married secretly and not tell your family?" He laughed like he always does and said, "Of course not. Do you think I'm going to get married and not tell you of all people?" But he's happy and that's the main thing. I often think of what he could have done on the football field if he had been able to stay healthy. And what a specimen of a man. Steve was a bit more stable with his relationships with women whereas I moved along pretty frequently.

The Marriott was a great place to work. I was there a number of years by now and what great times. Bill Skoglund, the big wheel in our region, who is the nicest guy you could ever meet, used to like to see some of the important people who came into the hotel to see me. Rico would come in regularly, or Andy Brickley, Lyndon Byers, Steve Bedrosian and Mark Whipple. Bill is a big fan of the Boston sports teams, as are his wife Beth and their kids; wonderful family, always making their way to see me no matter how busy they are. When he's bringing Mr. Bill Marriott around to the different properties, he would give me a "Hi, Dave" across the hallway even if Mr. Marriott's rushing him to go somewhere. People like that you love to see succeed. As a matter of fact, one of his daughters, Shannon, was playing softball and he asked me if I could help her with her hitting, which I did.

During Bill's tenure at our property, there was a girl who I started to date. She was one of the most attractive girls the hotel had seen in some time. Her name was Anastasia. I dated her for a while but broke it off after a short period of time. I liked her but at the time she was going through a divorce and I didn't want to deal with that. I know that's tough on someone. She came down after work one day and asked me why I've been avoiding her. I really didn't have an answer for her but we remained friends.

Dave Wallace, the longtime pitching coach of the Los Angeles Dodgers, was now becoming a friend of mine. Dave went to my alma mater, New Haven, years before me and was well known throughout baseball. One year out in California while visiting, I went to Dodger Stadium with Ralph Myerow. Dave was the pitching coach back then. I brought Ralph down and looked for Dave before a game. Sure enough, here he comes in from the bullpen area. I called to him and he made his way to us. I introduced myself and Ralph to him and said I pitched at New Haven after he did. He said he knew of me. Years ago, my cousin lived next to him in Rhode Island. She told him her cousin went to New Haven, as well. She said, "His name is Dave Caiazzo. Have you ever heard of him?" Dave responded, "I certainly have. He broke all my records there." What a pleasant man! People had told me that but once I met him, I saw that. We did get together a few times back in New England for dinner and different things. I got him to do a great talk on pitching for Eric Wedge and Mark Lombardi's Strike-One in Danvers. Talk about a nice person! Dave is the best, and probably one of the two or three best pitching coaches in baseball.

Steve's daughter Jenna is doing great. She landed a news reporter job in Carolina. She's exceptional at what she does. Time flies by.

Bobby Salamone, one of the good friends I played softball with after the baseball years, had some good observations over the years. "David," he'd ask. "With all the women I've seen you with over the years, why aren't you married?" I'd respond, "Bobby, maybe I want to live a nice, peaceful life with no stress or aggravation." That's the truth. That's how I feel.

A few years ago I thought I might change my opinion of what I had said to Bobby. A friend from work brought his girlfriend into work one day and she had a girlfriend of hers with her. I was introduced and the next day he asked me if I was interested in her. I told him I thought she was very attractive. Her name was Roseann, a nice Italian girl. She gave my friend her telephone number to give to me. I called and we went to Maine for a nice dinner on our first date. We dated regularly for more than a year and a half. I thought this might be the girl who was going to change my bachelor status. She had a beautiful condo in the seaport district in Boston. We did so much together, going to friends' parties, functions, just going out for dinners and events. We had fun. Coach V even came to Boston one night and he came out to dinner in the North End. He thought she was a great catch for me.

She was still modeling some. She was much younger than me but to be modeling after you are in your twenties is something. Roseann invited me to a time she was modeling at and she did a very nice job. She impressed me. Russ and Beth Hall came out with us a few times and thought she was going to be the one, also. Roseann would come to my baseball camp and take pictures. She really always wanted to be around me and I was getting to feel the same way about her. Mom, Joan and Steve liked her, as well. That was big. If they approved of her then I was heading in the right direction. She was talking about going to Italy some day with me. I was finding out she would always be looking out for me, whether I needed something to eat, or to stay warm, or getting some rest. She had all the ingredients for a nice wife some day. I knew that if she wasn't going to be my wife, then she at least was a great girl. I know Rocco would approve of Roseann if he were alive. Just prior to Roseann and I splitting up, she had written me a beautiful letter saying how in the last year and a half she had had the best time of her life and it's made her so happy. I felt terrible after that.

John Anquillare, one of the University of New Haven's all-time greats and first inductee into our hall of fame, left the school. He had been Coach V's assistant ever since Coach Tonelli retired some fifteen years prior. John was a tough guy who didn't put up with any bull crap. But he was a very good coach. You have to be when you coach under Coach V. When John finally left New Haven, he hooked on as the head baseball coach at the University of Bridgeport in Connecticut. Coach V was in his last season at the helm and John had asked me now that Coach V was leaving that I really had no obligation to be with New Haven any longer. He said, "Cai, why don't you join me and my staff?" I felt I still did have some obligation to New Haven but didn't want New Haven's new coach Raphael Cerrato looking over his shoulder all the time with a former player coaching under him. Cerrato had asked me to stay on as the special instructor.

So between trying to help John out and with Coach V leaving, I decided to go to Bridgeport with John. Coach V had told me that Raphael and the New Haven athletic director for years there wanted me to stay. Debbie Chin, the AD, was around a long time. I'll never forget years ago when Trixie was down Florida with the team, she told him to clean up his language around the pool at the hotel. Trixie used to talk and forget sometimes who was present.

33.

"Cai, You Go Through Women Like I Go Through Vodka"

COACH V HAD NOW COMPLETED his final year at the helm. What an illustrious career it was; the greatest, as I always said. No one better. He left as the top college coach of all time in winning percentage and second in wins. I'm sure if we weren't a school from New England, he would have been the leader in wins hands down. The only thing I regret was not being able to attend his 1000th victory. It was far away and something at work made it impossible for me to get there.

I attended and traveled to so many of his games over the years. Coach had put more than 100 players into pro ball So many people were so fond of him and there were those few who were jealous of him, as well. There are always the ones who are jealous. That's not a good thing to be.

When Coach V retired, I had a special necklace made for him. It was solid gold with white gold mixed in. It was a baseball with bats criss-crossed on it. It had his name on it and a quote from me on the back. He loved it but he certainly deserved it. What a coach but, more importantly, what a man! Everyone was waiting for his big retirement party and what a time it was. Hundreds of people attended and the guest speaker was Bobby Valentine, the great manager for the New York Mets and Texas Rangers. The other two speakers were Coach Tonelli and Coach Anquillare. The toastmaster was George Grande from ESPN sports and the voice of the New York Yankees and St. Louis Cardinals. It was the greatest banquet I have ever attended and I have been to some great ones. It was a great ending to a great career. Coach V mentioned me in his speech which made tears come to my eyes.

The University of New Haven was thinking of a date when it could officially retire legendary coach Porky Vieira's uniform, number 20. The announcement was made at the Hall of Fame dinner when Coach V was inducted. February 12, 2011 was the official date. I was really looking forward to this. It was being held in the school gymnasium and included the presentation and unveiling of his photo during halftime of a basketball game. I brought Roseann, who I was now back dating again. She knew Coach V from my camp in Malden three years ago, before she and I split up. She just loved him. I called Coach to let him know I would be there, of course, and that I would be taking Roseann. I wanted to make sure he remembered her. He did, of course, and said he really liked her. I told Coach not to mess up her name. He said, "Cai, you go through women like I do through vodka." He always has those great lines.

A lot of my ex-teammates and former players who I became very friendly with throughout the years also were going to be there. We had stayed in touch and were all looking forward to another great event. Debbie Chin, the New Haven athletic director, did a really nice job organizing the event. Roseann and I got there a little early because she had never seen my photo in the Hall of Fame section of the athletic building. She was very impressed. Then, on top of that, I was introducing her to many of my friends who are Hall of Famers so she was putting the plaques together with their pictures.

When Coach V walked in the first thing he did was ask where I was. When he found me, he pulled out a clementine orange out of his pocket and said, "Here, Cai, make sure you eat this." That's him, always looking out for me. They don't get any better than him. Over the years, though, I have given him moments of low blood sugars that put a scare into him, so I don't blame him for giving that to me.

Everyone packed into the gym, and everyone was spread out. Guys such as Tom Michalczyk, Dennis and Lenny Paglialunga, Pete Tranquillo, Bob Turcio, Don Murelli, Ronny Diorio, Coach John Anquillare and Coach Joe Tonelli. Coach Raphael Cerrato, who took over when Coach V retired, was great. A class guy who did a great job, winning more than thirty games a year ago. He just respects Coach V to the max and also respects all of the alumni and tries to stay in touch with everyone for different events.

While awaiting the big halftime show, Tom Michalczyk got my attention and said before he made it to the gym, he went to Sports Haven (a casino) and ran into one of our old teammates. He said this person didn't even know about Coach's event because no one knew how to get in touch with him for the last thirty years. Then he finally told me that person was "Keats," my old buddy who was my co-captain our senior year. I couldn't wait to see him. Tom had told him about the event and Keats asked who was going to be there. Tom told him a lot of the guys, and Cai will also be there. Tom said when Keats heard I was going to be there, his eyes opened wide and he said, "I'm going. I'll see you at the reception after the gym ceremony." I was just hoping he was coming. I couldn't wait to see him. I hadn't seen him in a little more than twenty years.

Halftime was now approaching. Everyone was excited. The PA announcer said, "Now is the time you've all been waiting for." He began to read all of Coach V's accomplishments as the baseball coach at New Haven. You can't believe his statistics; beyond belief. When Debbie Chin came out to introduce Coach V, the place erupted; a long, long standing ovation and, as Coach V only can do, he signaled everyone to sit down. For once, no one was listening to what he was saying. His huge picture on the gym wall was unveiled and everyone went crazy. When he took the microphone to speak, he said something I'll never forget. He said you're only as successful as your administration and your players. When he introduced Coach Tonelli, first he mentioned how great he was as an assistant to him. Then he said Coach Tonelli was responsible for getting guys like Bedrosian and Caiazzo to our program. I had tears in my eyes as he was talking. He had so many people who were greats at the school and he mentioned me with the former Cy Young Award winner and my good friend Steve Bedrosian. Then he mentioned both of us again. I looked at Roseann and she was as proud as I was. Coach did it again. Then Coach thanked John Anquillare, his other assistant coach, who I now work with at the University of Bridgeport. That was very nice. I was elbowing John to raise his hand so people would know where he was, but he didn't do it. John was proud, as well. Coach spoke for about five minutes and what a nice speech. Listening to him is always enjoyable.

The reception at the German Club across the street from the school was going to be great. When we got there, everyone was telling old baseball stories and the camaraderie among the players was something to see. Even Doc Basso, my very first roommate at New Haven, was there. We talked of the old days and it was fun. Everyone, and I mean everyone, loved Roseann when I was introducing her to them. After a short time, who do I see walking in but Tommy Keating (Keats). I ran over to him and we hugged each other as we both had huge smiles on our faces. Keats said, "Cai, when I heard you were going to be here, I said I'm going." He said he couldn't wait to see me. He kept telling me he loved me and he thinks of me all the time. I told him the same thing. We exchanged telephone numbers and said we would promise each other to stay in touch as he was coming to Boston to visit. We stayed at the bar and exchanged our old times together and we laughed and laughed.

We took many pictures and Roseann said what a wonderful bunch of friends and ex-teammates you have. I told her it all stems from Coach V. He has only good people he recruits. No bad people, only good ones. I, of course, before we left the gym, told Coach V I had something for him. He stopped in his tracks, smiled at me and said, "Vodka?" I told him I had a bottle of Absolute in the car for him.

After the great evening and entire day, we headed back to Boston. About ten minutes into our ride, Roseann turned to me and said, "David, I've never in my lifetime seen any one person so loved by everyone as you. I mean that. Never." I thanked her and told her the same thing I tell every-one. If you're good to people and they are good people as well, the con-nection will surface. We just have a great bond between all of us.

As the years were going by, I was the pitching coach at Austin Prep High School in Reading and was asked to work more consistently with Kenny Mazonson and the Malden Post 69 American Legion baseball team as their pitching coach. In addition, I was still working with the University of Bridgeport baseball team. Kenny Mazonson is just a lover of baseball. He coached Little League for many, many years and has been at the Post for better than twelve years. I would do anything for Kenny because he's a friend and has always been there for me when needed. I don't like to say "no" to anyone. If I do say "no", it's a good indication that I'm not a fan of that person.

There weren't many real good ballplayers at the Legion level but my job was to work with them and just try to teach them more and try to help them improve. Sometimes that was difficult. If they don't have the talent, there's not much you can do. I tried to help a few of the kids get into col-lege but most of the time they didn't have the grades or they didn't have the motivation to help themselves. A couple of kids, Ben Thomczyk for one, were pretty good. I got him into Bridgeport and really worked hard to get there. But once he got there, he needed to come back because the family needed him home. Ben was a real good kid and played as hard as he could for you. I liked that I pushed him but any competitive kid won't complain about a coach pushing him. There is no phoniness about me. People will always tell others, you'll know right from the get go if Dave Cai doesn't like you. I've said many times, if I don't like someone, I have trouble looking that person in the eye. No faking it with me.

The girls in my life would come and go. Most of the time because I would not commit but on one occasion I was lucky. I liked both of these girls at one period of time. I don't remember if I was very low with my blood sugar or not when I invited both girls to a summer game I was pitching. This one girl came to the game and was there about four innings. I kept looking over at her and she'd smile at me if I gave her a glance. Then she sent someone over to me to say she wasn't feeling good and had to leave but for me to call her after the game. No sooner did she leave, than I see the other girl I forgot I invited coming into the park. She walked right past the other girl leaving. She stayed until the end and waited for me. That would have been quite a scene had they both been there at the same time. I lucked out.

So many times now as I am coaching the Legion players, I am at the same field (Devir Park) where I used to be on the mound looking out into the Fellsway for my father. After he'd leave work in Boston, he'd jump on the subway to make sure he didn't miss me pitch. Sometimes he'd get there just after the game had started or other times by the second inning. But I never felt 100 percent comfortable until Dad was there. As soon as I saw him, I was at ease. It brings back great memories.

Some of my friends comment on how I love the attention of the exposure I got but honestly I just wanted to be a ball player, not just a normal one but an exceptional one. And as far as getting the extra attention, if you are performing at a high level then the celebrity part of that automatically comes with it.

Trixie's mother had taken ill at this time and they didn't give her much time to live. She finally passed away and another fine woman had gone. She was a wonderful lady who treated me with the utmost respect all the time. When Trixie's father was alive years ago, we'd all sit down and talk sports or really anything. It was fun. We had some great Trixie stories. The one that comes to mind is the time Trixie borrowed Bobby Orr's van. Trixie worked at the Massachusetts Treasury and often used to pick up Bobby Orr for Treasurer Bob Crane. We had all planned to go see the Harvard-Yale football game in New Haven and hook up with some of my old buddies. We had about six or seven of us going. So rather than take two cars, Trixie said he wanted to ask Bobby Orr if we could take his van. It was brand new, maybe a month or two old. I said, "Do you think he's going to let you?" Trixie said, "He might." Trixie was right; Bobby said yes. The night before, Trixie was to go to Weston where Bobby lived to pick up the van. It was a

Friday evening and I was resting on the couch. I heard the doorbell ring and my father went down to answer the door. I heard him say, "Hi, Trixie." Trixie said, "Mr. Cai, is Dave around?" My father said, "Yes, but he's resting. Let me get him up." Trixie said, "Tell him to hurry." That didn't sound good.

When I went downstairs, Trixie said, "Dave, come here." When I went over to the van, I said it's beautiful. He said, "Yeah, look over here." He pointed to a big damaged area. I said, "What happened?" He said an eighty-eight-year-old man cut him off on the Expressway. Prior to this, all of the guys figured it would cost us about $18 each for food, gas, tickets, etc. The next day when we met everyone before we got on the road, Trix told everyone what happened. But he said, "Now, instead of everyone's fee being $18, it's going to be $800. Everyone practically went after Trixie. He was funny. We helped out but it all worked out. A year or two later, I ran into Bobby at a time at the Copley Plaza and when he came to the desk, I said, "Hi, Bobby." He greeted me and smirked and said, "Dave you guys were bombed that night with my van, weren't you?" I told him honestly what happened. He said, "I'm only kidding. I don't care." What a great person he is. Everything you hear about him is true.

I was missing the competitiveness of playing baseball now that I wasn't pitching any more. After watching the teams in the league for a few years I retired, I noticed the talent just wasn't there. Pitchers not making quality pitches and with less velocity and command. The infielders not making routine plays and outfielders botching fly balls. As I was watching teams, you would hear things like "Oh, they retired so and so's number last year or this team retired their guy so and so after twelve years. I don't care how long a guy has played, he still has to have been exceptional for anyone to retire his number. God, Eddie Larson, from our great Augustine's teams, said to me recently, "Cai, your number twenty-one, Joe DiSarcina's number and Freddy Campatelli's number were retired." We just didn't have a big shindig about it but if you noticed, those three numbers were never issued again. No one had worn them since we left. You can't have mediocrity for stats and have your number retired.

34.

Johnny V And Harry, Both Dead!

IN THE LAST YEAR OR so, two of my dear friends and teammates passed away, Harry Mehos and John Valeri. Harry Mehos may be the most loyal ever to be involved in the local sports scene. Harry was with me in high school and the Intercity League for more than fifteen years. I drove him to every Intercity League Augustine's A's game for years. He was a breath of fresh air. What a kid. We had more laughs over the years. Harry, for some reason, used to refer to himself as Starsky and me as Hutch. They were the stars from the Starsky and Hutch TV show years ago. I'd be on the mound and Harry would yell out, "Let's go, Hutch" or something like that. Whatever Harry wanted to call me was fine with me. Harry was the man.

Johnny Valeri, my teammate in junior college, the University of New Haven and Augustine's Athletics, was the other person who passed away. Johnny was the nicest guy. He was one year behind me at school so when we were at Mass. Bay together and I left to go to New Haven, John followed there the next year. Then I helped him hook on with our Augustine's team. John did a great job. It was strange how I found out about Johnny not feeling well. I got a call one day at work from a good guy I played with one season, Billy Dunn. He said, "Cai, you played with John Valeri, didn't you?" I said, "Yes, why?" He told me he heard John only had a short time to live. That shocked me. I immediately called a couple of the guys but no one had heard anything.

A couple of weeks went by and our Legion team was getting ready to start a game. The umpire, Joe, turned to me and said, "Cai, one of your players is chewing tobacco." I told the kid to take it out of his mouth because you cannot chew any more. The umpire went over to the kid and told him that chewing wasn't any good for anyone. He said his close friend only had a couple of days to live because he had throat cancer. This story sounded familiar so I said, "Joe, who are you talking about." He said, "One of my close boyhood friends but you wouldn't know him." I said, "Who?" He answered by saying "John Valeri." I said, "I wouldn't know him? I played on three teams with him and lived with him one year at New Haven. What are you talking about?"

A week or so later, John died. What a great kid he was. John always used to say something to me because he knew how much my arm injury hurt. "Cai, you're amazing. You go out there every time you're scheduled to pitch and go the distance every time," he said. "I don't know how you do it."

I had ended my summer camp a couple of years ago after twenty-seven years. That was a long time. We had some great times and some great people who worked for me. But the bottom line was we helped develop a lot of kids. I was very proud of that. Years ago I had a nice conversation with the great singer Joan Baez. When she would check into the Copley Plaza she would always come over to me and she invited me to have a glass of wine with her a few times. I never had the wine but I would stop by her room and we talked about my involvement with baseball. She would say, "I just think its wonderful you help the kids like you do. We need more of that." She was a very nice lady and enjoyable to talk to.

When I think of the old Copley Plaza hotel, I think of so many great incidents that happened. One of the interesting ones was when Yul Brynner checked in. I had to go to his room for something he needed. I remember the first year he checked in he was with his maid, an Asian girl. The next year he came back in and his maid was now his wife.

Another time Gloria Swanson, a famous actress from the days of silent movies, checked in. She was very old and she went out for a breath of fresh air. When she came back in, she asked me to help her get into her bed because it was elevated some. I helped her and always like to tell that story.

So many memories and so much that remains in my mind. For so many years, Mom and Dad were so proud of their children. I'll tell everyone, no one could be prouder of my parents than we are of them. Just yesterday, I went to Dad's grave. It would have been his ninety-first birthday. It was cold but I stayed for fifteen minutes alone just thinking of what a great father he was and how wonderful he brought us up and took care of Mom. I didn't bring any flowers because Mom always says, "Don't bring flowers in the cold weather because they'll just die or someone will steal them. Dad always said to sprinkle a little red wine on the grave. That I did. It must be an Italian tradition. I was thinking "The greatest man ever."

Just a few months ago I decided to resign from scouting. Eighteen years was enough. All the traveling, trying to get the proper information and project someone's potential. Someone years ago said something that made sense. He said potential means "you haven't done shit." So true. But to do all that work so someone above you can cash in, instead of the person who deserves the credit, is ludicrous. But those people will know exactly who they are when they look in the mirror. As it turns out, those people are not involved in baseball any longer nor should they be. Coach V, the smartest baseball man I ever knew, said it a year or so ago. He said, "These scouts don't know what they're talking about. They're trained to press the radar gun and press the stop watch and that's it. Anybody can do that stuff. It's being able to identify a kid's makeup and what he has inside. Yes, you do need to have the ability to run, throw, hit, etc. But I've seen kids who can do that but can't perform under pressure or get the money hit when it counts or win that ball game when it counts. Some of these scouts were and are car salesmen or in the oil business."

Coach says, "Cai, after talking to them, I don't know where they are coming from but after talking to you I feel I've just had a great baseball conversation." The people who are always trying to pull you down usually don't go too far in life themselves. And as far as my friends all know "You can't get Dave to stoop to their level. Dave is on top of his game." Most of these scouts, as it turned out, never even put on a uniform let alone played the game. I was amazed to find out. It's really sad. But anyone who was trying to get the better of me lost out. They may have picked up a few dollars more but lost their jobs in the process and, most importantly, they lost a good friend. Enough said on that subject.

Now, I know I have great friends. Russell's father (Charlie) passed away a few months ago. Charlie was a good guy. He always called me his son. Everything started to deteriorate on Charlie leading to his death. Charlie's wife died many years ago. She was a wonderful wife and a great mother to Russ and his sister Lorraine. I know Russell was crushed when she died. Russell is just one of those good guys and married a great girl in his wife Beth. They have a great marriage and I was very proud when Russ asked me to be his best man when they were married. That was a great wedding and Charlie was so happy to see Russ marry such a great girl in Beth. I know Russ' mom would have been just as proud if she were alive. He's just a loyal friend. I can't remember him missing many of my games when I pitched. He loved to watch with my Dad.

Ralph Suarez, from Philly, informed me of his son Richie's sickness. He has a form of leukemia. I feel so bad for his family. Ralph's another one of my close friends who would do anything for you. Just a down-to-earth great guy. We had so many laughs and also some tough times in the minors. Ralph and his lovely wife Denise have a close-knit family and I certainly hope everything turns out for the better for Richie. When Ralph called me to give me the news, the first thing I told him was how Steve Bedrosian's son Cody had the same illness at a younger age and he pulled through. I know that gave Ralph some positive feedback that leukemia can be beat.

35.

I Persevered And Came Out On Top

I'M AT A GREAT PLACE with the Marriott. Work is enjoyable and the people I work with make it special. The guests can be difficult at times but you have to keep smiling even if they're upset with something. I went to school for this years ago and now have been in the business since 1978. Our general manager Victor Aragona is easy to work for. He goes about his business in a professional manner and keeps an upbeat attitude, no matter what. Treats me with respect and that's important.

Lauren Bartkus and Cora Genas from human resources are wonderful people. Cora I've known since I first started at the hotel when I was the garage manager. She would come to my office and we would talk for hours. Great girl and a Virgo like me. She has that electric smile that catches your eye. She always makes her way to me to tell me, "Dave, you're just a regular guy. You just treat everyone with respect."

Randy Arpea is now the assistant general manager. Randy is my guy as far as talking each day, having lunch or whatever area of the hotel we're in. We can small talk. It doesn't have to be about work. I got to know Randy's family pretty well in the last few years. His wife Lori is just the nicest person. They have two beautiful daughters Mia and Noelle. Lori always finds a way to send me something I'm able to eat with my wheat problem. I don't know how many times she has sent things to me through Randy. Randy and Lori are bringing the kids up very well. They are the most well-behaved kids you will see.

Every morning Randy, as well as Victor, make sure they find their way to me to say good morning or just talk a little baseball. And our front office manager Ryan Tavares does a great job, as well. Ryan and I get along great and he's a super guy. We are both Yankee fans, as well, so we talk quite a bit outside of work-related issues

Just like baseball, if you generally don't like playing for the manager, you are not going to perform up to par. I really enjoy my job.

So often I look back and wish I had settled down with one of the women I dated. The Arpea family is one I look at and say if I settle down some day that is a family I wish mine would be like.

I was too hard on evaluating people and often times would say one of the women wouldn't make a good wife or mother. Just thinking of that would make me go the other way. And I'm sure I was wrong on quite a few of them.

Another woman I think of was from Florida. I met her while coaching at New Haven. While down south on our spring trip, she came to our games. I would ask who she was and one of the coaches told me she was an aunt of one of the players. Her name was Yvonne. What a knockout! I found my way to her one day and we hit it off pretty good. She finally invited me to go out with her at one of the restaurants in the nearby area. She had that Italian look to her with the dark hair and beautiful smile. One night she asked me to take a ride to meet her close to where she lived. I was a little tired so I asked Trixie to take the ride with me. When we got to the restaurant, we had a great time at the bar. After a couple of hours, we made our way outside. I told Trixie to meet me back at the car so I could walk Yvonne back to her car. I told Trixie he didn't need the keys because the car was open. It was a cold night for Florida. So when I got to Yvonne's car we quickly went in and did a little fooling around. I kept thinking of Trixie waiting for me. I said to Yvonne "he's gonna kill me." It must have been a good ninety minutes or so I kept him waiting.

Finally, Yvonne and I called it a night. However, when she drove me back to the car, I figured Trixie would be inside sleeping by now. As we approached, we saw Trixie standing outside the car with his teeth chattering. I got out and said, "I'm sorry, Trix. What are you doing out here?" He said, "The car door was locked." I laughed for the whole trip back to our hotel. We got into a big argument. I said, "Lighten up." He didn't want to hear me. I don't blame him. We were both so mad he called me "bush league." I said, "What do you know about being bush league." He said, "Nothing 'til I met you." Good line. We laugh to no end to this day about that. But at the time he was mad!

Yvonne even went way out of her way to meet me at the airport when we were leaving Florida. She looked great that day. But, in all honesty, she looked great every day. We stayed in touch for a few years. But that long-distance romance doesn't work out well. She would have been a great wife and mother.

Another girl I thought could have been a nice wife was an airline stewardess my sister-in-law Donna set me up with. Her name was Diane. A few years before I took her out she was dating Joe Montana. She said I reminded her of him. I got that one quite a bit during Joe's playing days. She was originally from Pennsylvania but now was working out of Boston. What kind of got me to drift away from her was when she told me she eventually wanted to move back home to Pennsylvania. I had no urge whatsoever to move to Pennsylvania.

I know Lisa Pagliarulo would have made the perfect mate for me. I know her family very well and just know what type of family they are. All good people, from the parents all the way down to the kids, and their kids, as well. When I would get a bit nervous talking or even calling someone, I knew that person was special. Each time I would attempt to call Lisa, I would get a chill of excitement in my body. That told me something. Too bad I wasn't persistent enough to follow through more with the ones I should have.

Wayne, one of the long-time associates at the bell stand at Long Wharf Marriott said to me recently, "Dave, I've never seen so many beautiful girls come in with you over the years. I said, "Not so much recently, Wayne." He said, "I used to look forward to you coming in because whoever you were with was going to be something to see." I used to think there would always be someone out there to outdo the ones I was with. Someone better-looking somewhere waiting for me to find them. I found out that wasn't necessarily true. I wanted everyone to say when they saw me out with one of the girls, "Dave Cai was with the best-looking girl at the party or at the event or at the banquet, whatever." I don't think like that any more. Those days are over.

As I look back, the women with the biggest heart are the ones I should have been more concerned with. Carole was always looking out for me. I remember days of my camp, when her son Michael was attending it. I put in some long, tough days and would not even slow down one minute. At camp's end, I would be wiped out. Carole would always be there to pick up her son, most of the time while she was working. She'd be in her police car. She would notice me being so low with my blood sugar that I would almost be unconscious. She was so concerned about me that she didn't want me to drive home from the park. Of course, I won the argument so she would follow me home in the police car, making sure I was escorted home. She was always showing concern for me. I always appreciated that. What a caring girl! Not only was she good-looking but also had a heart of gold to go with it. Once I got home, she made her way into my house to let my mother know of the state of mind I was in. She loved my mother and my mother loved her. She would alert my mother if I needed some orange juice immediately or some food very quickly. As I remember, she did this a few times. I was just so stubborn sometimes with my diabetes, I wouldn't allow anyone to help me. Just once again, the nature of the disease. I just wouldn't allow anyone to get into my world, so to speak. Even with my family and closest friends.

After all the years that had passed, Lynda from Medicine Hat, Canada, wanted to meet with me. She knew I was going to Florida with the University of New Haven to instruct once again on their southern trip. We decided she was going to make the long trip. Trixie made that trip as well because he was on pretty good terms with Coach V. As soon as we got checked in and got settled in our rooms, Lynda called and waited for us in the lobby. She traveled with her sister Maureen. They were two good-looking women. Lynda was a sight for sore eyes, as my father used to say. We all went to the lounge and met up with Coach V and Coach Tonelli for some appetizers and drinks. Drinks were a given with Coach V in the vicinity. I had a small gift for Lynda. So we weren't in the lounge long when we went back to my room. One thing led to another and we didn't get back to the lounge for about two hours. When we did get back to everyone in the lounge, Coach V was all over me with some of his one-liners. We laughed and laughed. It was great to see Lynda again and we spent a lot of time together. She stayed in Florida for about six days. When we were alone, she would tell me how she dreamed of being with me again. She knew how she could satisfy me in bed and she was a great girl besides all that. When she was ready to go back to Canada, she cried quite a bit. I was sad to see her leave, as well.

After the spring trip, it was back to work, lessons and coaching back in Boston. One day while working in front of the Marriott Long Wharf, I was having a conversation with a couple of the valets. Then I heard one of the valets say, "Here comes one for you, Davey." When I looked up, this beautiful girl with the nicest-looking legs you ever saw, was walking toward us. She approached us and looked scared. She said, "Did anyone see a tow truck tow a car from across the street?" I answered "no" but offered to help find out what happened. I went into my manager's office and began to call the Boston Police to see who to call. They gave me a telephone number. When I called, sure enough, they had the car in a very bad section of Dorchester. She said, "I'm scared to go to that part of town by myself." I told her, "Don't worry, I'll see if I can leave work for a little while to go with you."

I checked with my boss and he said "that's fine." I drove her and her name was Kristy. The car was in a dangerous area, no doubt. But we got her car for her. She said, "I don't know how to thank you enough. What a gentleman." I couldn't have imagined her going there by taxi and dealing with them in that area. She used to tell people that I was her "knight in shining armor." We stayed in touch after that. She was striking. As it turned out, she was a Harvard grad and was a model and actress. She was very talented. She lived in Charlestown behind the U.S.S. Constitution in a nice, small apartment. We started to date some. She gave a great body massage, I remember. Then she would always say I'm going to give you a hand massage. When she finished, I was so relaxed. It reminded me of when my father used to give me massages. But his were even better because they were firm and he had those big, strong hands.

Kristy would travel quite a bit. When she came back to Boston after she left the area for a while, she would stay with me at my place. A few times we took trips to Maine and New Hampshire to meet friends of hers, and mine, as well. We spent a lot of time together. Years later, she moved to California and I would go out to the West Coast and meet at her place in Laguna Beach and then go out quite often. The first time I slept with her wasn't until I went out to California, believe it or not. To this day, she still calls and invites me to California with an open invitation.

The great thing about playing professionally is you bond with so many people. I always would say it's not the on-the-field activities you miss as much as the locker room and night activities. You miss that camaraderie with the players. But you keep the friendships. So many of the players I played with or met along the way would come to Boston when playing the Red Sox; players such as Julio Franco or Joe Cowley or Mike Raczka. I would meet up with them and we would be happy to see each other. Whether they called ahead of time to tell me when they'd be in town or me calling them to find out when they would be in. I would pick them up and go into Daisy Buchanan's in Boston or back to my Pub or just anywhere for good conversation while having dinner or lunch. That's friendship. One time Franco came in and I fixed him up with my attorney friend and they liked each other. I would go to a Cleveland-Red Sox game or a Texas Rangers-Red Sox game and bring either a girl friend or a few of my buddies. My attorney, Rose, really liked Julio and would always ask me when he would be coming into town.

I used to crack up with the softball guys. They're playing softball for a reason. They couldn't play the big game. It was much faster, you had to be quicker, you had to have a much better arm, be a better fielder, be an all-around athlete. One of my best friends, Bobby Salamone, was a lifetime softball player. He was pretty good. But I used to tease him that he wouldn't be able to play baseball. He is a great guy. I gave him the nickname "Surfin' Sal" when I played with him for a few years. He loved that name. We still call him "Surfin'" to this day. But, I've never seen a guy love softball as much as he does. He lived, slept, and drank softball. He is an Everett guy. Almost everyone from that city played softball. Most of them thought they were playing pro baseball. "Surfin'" wasn't like that, though. I couldn't understand what those guys were thinking. One time there was a big benefit softball game at Everett Stadium. I was invited to play. There were guys such as former Celtics players John Havlicek and Hank Finkel, former Bruins Ken Hodge, Gerry Cheevers and John Bucyk, people like that. A lot of the Everett softball players got to play, naturally. I remember being on deck to hit and while I was taking some practice swings, one of the Everett guys who thought he was good came up to me. He said, "I'm going to hit in front of you." I was furious when he said that. I turned to him and said, "Get behind me. People aren't here to see you play." He got the message and hit after me. That really got me ticked off. He was one of those guys who was out of shape, overweight and didn't even resemble a ballplayer to anyone. I don't know what he was thinking. Some people are told only by their friends or family that they're great and somehow they honestly believe it. But that won't happen outside of those people who aren't legitimate people themselves.

Coach V used to say to me, "Cai, you just keep doing what you do. You do it the way it's supposed to be done." I think I know what he meant. No phoniness, no put ons or kissing up to anyone. I never had to. People just know that's Davey Cai! I never tried to kiss my way to be a high type of executive or call someone who may have a lot of money and ask him for a job. That's not me I know many people who have so much money but not once have I asked any of them to help me along in life. It goes back to the old saying that if no one is telling you how good you are then you usually start telling people how good you are. As I become older, I really despise arrogance. There is nothing that gets me riled up more than if someone doesn't say hello to you when they walk by or they show that look of confidence when everyone knows they have none. Show me that confidence all you want but if you haven't done anything in life, I don't want to hear it. Bend someone else's ear.

When I was diagnosed with celiac disease a few years ago, it was so difficult to deal with. People didn't understand. It really can affect the diabetes to a great extent. If I go off my diet with the celiac, it can aggravate the diabetes. So many times I felt like collapsing either in work or outside my job.

But never complained. People would annoy me and I might be aggressive on my end but no one would ever know why. I would check my blood sugar and see it is either 40 or 400. That can bring on a big change in behavior. No one keeps themselves in better shape than I do so you know it's going to happen sooner or later that you've hit a real low or high and it will really get you dazed or sometimes laid out. The danger can occur if you have diabetes and have a low while driving the car. So many times that happened to me. One night I was driving home from work and I was the second car at a red light. The light changed three times before I decided to go around. As I looked in, a woman was almost keeled over the steering wheel. I pulled over. I figured something serious was wrong. When I opened the car door, she was very unstable and almost unconscious. I had some fruit and chocolate in my car so I ran over to get some. I gave it to her. I asked her if she was diabetic and I wasn't surprised to hear that she was. When she started to come around with the food in her system, I told her to move over and I pulled the car to the side of the road and stayed with her for about thirty minutes. When I saw she was able to drive, I asked her some questions and she was fine. I know I would have liked someone to do that for me had that been me in that situation. She was so appreciative. I got her telephone number when she said she was fine and didn't need me to follow her home. I called her home and spoke with her husband and he thanked me over and over again. It made me feel great to be able to help that woman.

I don't know how else to explain what living with diabetes is like other than saying it's like living on the edge. Death feels like it is so close at times. You can feel so great at times and other times like you aren't going to live another hour. So many times I explain to people you just don't go a full day feeling good. The entire day you can say "that was a great day, I felt good at least ten or twelve hours of it."

One day traveling back from an event at New Haven, I came as close to death as I could possibly feel. While traveling through the Mass. Turnpike tunnel, I was so low with my blood sugar count, I must have pulled the steering wheel too hard switching lanes. I veered off so fast, my vehicle was going completely sideways. I was only a couple of feet from the wall when I started to turn the steering wheel back and forth. I don't know how it happened but the vehicle's front and back side were swinging back and forth but it finally straightened out. My heart was in my mouth but God must have been with me again. I was going approximately seventy miles an hour so I would have been killed. When I straightened the car out, I went to the next lane and was looking in my rear view mirror to see what cars were around me. I noticed about four or five behind me that slowed down, probably thinking I was drunk, and not wanting to get near me. As I now was going about fifty miles an hour, cars were passing me slowly and as I looked at each one of them, people would be asking me if I was OK. I would give them the thumbs up sign. Wow, was I lucky! My life went right by me on this one.

One day while painting my house, I was getting very low with my blood sugar count. But, as usual, I continued to finish the job instead of getting something to eat in my system. Russell happened to stop by to visit and said, not more than five minutes later, "Have you eaten anything?" He said I was extremely low and for us to go get something to eat. Being as low as I was, of course I was stubborn, maybe more than usual. I kept saying I was alright. Russ said I was getting so bad that he tried to hold me up as I was starting to lose my balance. He said he didn't realize how strong I was until he tried to pull me away to go with him. He said he couldn't budge me. My body was so out of balance, I was swaying. I felt it but your mind doesn't work in synch with your body. I finally went with Russ but it was a struggle for me, and for Russ, as well. Only Russ would stay with me as he did, not letting me stay like that and eventually try to make it home on my own by car and possibly endanger myself or others. Other friends and family would have done the same for me but Russ, I guess you might say, is always there for me. He is just a great guy.

Another incident involved an old high school classmate of mine who had an incredible body and was very attractive, as well. She kept pursuing me over the years, then finally she and I said "let's get it going." She arranged, at least a week in advance, for us to meet at a hotel on Route One in Saugus. This was her idea from the get go. Of course, that sounded great to me. She made the reservation and paid in advance. It was a Friday night and I was to meet her at 6 p.m. My day, however, wasn't going well from early morning on. I remember getting backed up in time plus didn't have enough time to get something to eat beforehand. That was, once again, my fault. I should always make time for that. I was just trying to get to her by a reasonable hour. I was seeing two of everything. My blood count had to be, it seemed, about 35 or 40. That's not good. By the time I got to the hotel it was about 7 p.m. Kathy had brought food for both of us and was dressed really sexy. Unfortunately, the state I was in wasn't going to allow me to enjoy the food or the sex. I could not perform and I was as disappointed as she was but that was one of those bad diabetes days. Kathy, I remember, jumped in bed within ten minutes of the time we got there but that didn't seem to work even with the great outfit she was in. I remember almost falling asleep on her. I was so low by the time I got to her that the food we ate wasn't going to bring my blood sugar up to normal. Too bad. She was a good girl and I knew we both were looking forward to a good night.

36.

One Last Standing Ovation

AS TIME GOES ON, YOU never forget the good people you come across in your lifetime. Unfortunately, you don't forget the bad people, either. One incident I'll never forget was one of my last games pitching in the Intercity League; a game at Arlington against the Arlex Oilers. My arm was about a sore as I ever experienced it. I pitched into the last inning and won the game 1-0. I started to tire at the very end of the game. I didn't want to come out but Johnny Brickley came out to me and said, "Great job, Cai. You got us right where we wanted you to get us," and then he took me out for the last two outs. When I came out, the entire crowd who were in the grandstands stood up and gave me a standing ovation. I think they knew that might be the end of the line for me. That was so nice. Great feeling. I'll tell you, the game can give such heartaches but also so much joy.

Bridgeport University is now the school I've been working with. One of the first kids I helped go there was a boy named Derek Cotoni. I got him a full scholarship. He had a pretty good career. He's been graduated now for two years but to this day he still refers to me as Mr. Caiazzo, and his mother is so nice. She sends me letters each year thanking me for what I did for Derek. She also sends me several gift certificates at Christmas every year. What a nice, nice family and so respectful. That's the way a boy is supposed to be brought up. His mother should be so proud of him. He'll do well in life. I know it. The key to his, or anyone's, success is hard work.

To get rewarded, you must be patient. If you have success in life, whether it is in business or sports, you must have the ability to wait. If you have success in sports, the rewards will come eventually. If you have a great career in high school, the hall of fame will be in the future; the same in college or the major leagues. If you have a great season, the all-scholastic awards, post-season awards, etc., will follow at the season's end. Post-season awards don't come to anyone who hasn't had a great season. I used to tell guys over the years not to be too happy after one outstanding game. You have to have continuous success game after game. Steve and I in the Caiazzo family had that quality. We were very proud of that. My thought was always not to put your fate in the hands of someone who isn't qualified to do it, or in the hands of anyone at all. At work, I never wanted someone who wasn't qualified to give me a review on my performance. They shouldn't be in that position. The same goes for an umpire at a lower level of the game. If you give the umpire the option to call pitches, balls that are strikes, then that's not right. I want to win the game myself without having to rely on someone to help me. That's the way I've always felt. I tell the same thing to my pitchers that I coach now. If I get on a kid about a team putting too much contact to his pitches, he might say, "Well, Coach, Johnny at shortstop or Jimmy at second base should have had those balls." You know what I tell them, "That's bullshit. You let them hit the ball. You don't have to worry if you don't have that contact being made. That's your fault."

The coaching part of the game is different in today's era. Today you have to handle kids with kid gloves. They are more sensitive, not as tough, and have a disposition about them that I can't believe at times. I tell the kids today that they wouldn't last one day even if they had the talent to play for Coach Vieira or Tom Zimmer. Vieira would tear them to shreds. These kids today would not be able to take it. They would quit or be so paranoid that they wouldn't be able to perform. Back in the day, Coach V would blast you but he knew you would be able to take it to some degree. He would say, "Once I stop noticing you, that's when you have to start worrying because it means I stopped believing in you." Coaches have to be held to a higher standard. They can't be anyone who is unprofessional or full of bull. They have to be someone who the players look up to and respect. You can't ask for respect; you earn respect. I'll go to my grave knowing I get my respect from people for the way I conduct myself and how I performed between those lines and off the field. Years ago, I used to tell a buddy of mine that it doesn't matter how you die but how each one of us lived our lives. People question the way they lived their lives, as they look back, all the time. That I never did. I have no regrets and couldn't have asked for a better life. I remember going in for an interview with an athletic director for a baseball job years ago. I remember him asking me how I could stand all the atten-

tion I constantly got. I really didn't think about it much. I responded by saying, "Mickey Mantle wasn't happy with the way he lived his life but Dave
Caiazzo is."

I never forgot the people who made an impact on my life; Frank Adorn,
Russ Hall, John "Trixie" Trischitta, Frank Vieira, Mo Maloney, Don
Murelli, Ralph Suarez, Steve Ring, Fla Strawn, Mac Singleton, Rico Petrocelli, Lou DiSanto and Steve Bedrosian and so many others, without having to mention my family, of course.

No matter who or what tried to take me out, I persevered and came out
on top. None of my family or friends would attempt to, but there are plenty
of people out there who would try. But I learned a long time ago, you can't
give anyone any reason to do so or any ammunition to work with. My father
would always say there are a lot of bad people who try to bring you down
to their level. You can't let it happen. I found out Dad was right. He usually
was. He was always ahead of his time.

Meeting so many great people over the years I think helped to mold me
in the right direction. Classy people is what I like to see. I'll never forget the
trip I made to California a few years ago when I met the Price is Right's
Bob Barker and the late Rod Roddy backstage with former girlfriend
Christina, and that same day meeting Dian Parkinson backstage. And on
that same trip meeting Michael Jackson's wife Debbie Rowe at a restaurant.
They were all so nice to me. They showed the class I expect to see when
meeting these famous people. You never want to walk away saying those
people aren't what you expected or that they were not friendly.

When I met Don Zimmer (Tom's dad) at Fenway Park immediately
after our season ended in 1978. He was the nicest guy. I told him Tom
wanted me to meet him so he expected me. Real classy person. You want
people to turn out the way you expect or anticipate them to be like. At least
in the good sense, not bad. Red Sox manager Joe Morgan was another good
guy when I met him at a banquet; very friendly and outgoing. Eric Wedge,
former Cleveland Indians manager whose facility in Danvers is where I
now give my private pitching lessons, is nothing more than a top-notch guy.
Always going out of his way to say "hello" to me whether he's busy or not.
I brought Dave Wallace, the former Red Sox pitching coach to do a clinic
at the facility. Dave is also a good friend of mine He's a former University
of New Haven righthanded pitcher as well. He played for Coach V a few
years before my time. We hit it off the first time I met Dave at Dodger Stadium when he was the pitching coach for them a few years ago. What a true
professional!

Joe Cowley, former Yankees and White Sox pitcher, is another great guy. He and I hit it off right away at Steve Bedrosian's wedding. He's one of those fun-loving guys who is very personable and loves to go out and have a drink or two but never gets past the "OK, that's enough for me tonight" point. Joe and Kimberly (Joe's wife) invited me to their wedding years ago but I couldn't make it. But Joe and I stayed in touch pretty consistently over the years.

All of these guys are just some of the great people in the game who I've become friends with. There are so many more but these are some of the rewards you encounter while being in the game of baseball. The other day, I ran across a friend of mine I haven't seen in a couple of years. We talked for quite a while. "Davey," he said. "You haven't changed a bit. Stay like you are. Someone I was talking to about you recently said the same thing. He also said you'll never see Dave Cai with bad people. He knows who to choose as friends." I love hearing those remarks. I won't lower myself to someone else's standards. I have too much pride!

Some of the people in today's era call themselves hitting or pitching coaches. From what I have seen, nothing could be further than the truth. There is this guy I never heard of before who claimed to be a hitting coach and was having a lot of the local kids play for the team he organized and coached. He was charging parents huge money and they were getting nothing back in return; no exchange of knowledge of the game. This guy knew practically next to nothing. I watched him one day do a hitting session with each kid on his team at Trum Field in Somerville. What a comedy! Without exaggeration, I must have watched him for at least 40 minutes and he didn't say anything to any of the hitters while they were hitting. I noticed numerous things kids were doing wrong but he never corrected them. I mean, not one word! If he did say something, it had no meaning or substance. After I spoke with him on the telephone one day for at least an hour, I realized this guy was a fraud. I could never do that. When I work with someone, whether it's pitching or just talking baseball, they walk away knowing they learned something.

A friend of mine named Lori from Revere always reminds me how her sons both learned so much from me. Lori had great interest in her boys and wants them to learn the correct way. Let's not forget, I saw the great Vieira teaching hitting for years, and then what I learned throughout the years from professionals on pitching. I never had, and won't, tolerate being just "good." I have a passion for what I do, whether it was softball when I played after my baseball career, or whatever it was, I took it seriously. Dana Brown, the principal at Malden High, and former softball teammate, said something interesting. Dana tells people that "if you put Cai in an open field in softball, he'd hit .800." Dana is now a real, good friend. But that's the way I played, hard all the time. Dana, himself, was a pretty good pitcher in softball and was just a great guy and teammate. I just respect those guys like him who are "regular" guys.

37.

Lifelong Memories With No Regrets

AFTER ALL THESE YEARS I still miss Rocco dearly. After seeing what some families go through and how kids are treated by their dads, I cherish the childhood I had even more. What a man! He was what we call a man's man. Greatest man I ever knew. Knew how to bring up a family; stressed the important things in life; always showed a tremendous interest in our lives. Dad didn't have a lot of money but he took care of his family the best way he knew how and that was good enough for me and all the Caiazzos. When he walked into a room, he electrified that room. His good looks didn't hurt his presence either. He could talk with anyone. Oftentimes I laugh to myself when I think of a time behind our Pub on Pearl Street. After closing the Pub one night, I ended up with this girl after hours. We ended up in my car in the back parking lot. We both fell asleep but somehow I woke up and got into the front seat. I wasn't in the front seat for more than a couple of minutes when Rocco knocked on the window and said, "Dave, you beat me here today. I can't believe it." See, no one got up as early as Dad in the morning. He thought I was opening up that morning and couldn't believe I beat him there. But he never noticed the girl practically naked in the back seat. He said "I'll see you inside" and left. I still can't believe he missed that one. I would have been really embarrassed if he had seen that. But when I think back, he probably wouldn't have said anything to me' maybe a "just be careful."

Everyone in the Caiazzo household is happy and well. Mom is amazing, still looking like she's about 60 years old. Steve, Joan all happy. That's important to me. All the things as a family we experienced together; the

Kennedy assassination probably the biggest and most historic event anyone could ever live through.

No doubt, though, was Rocco's death, saddest day in all our lives. So many of the things that went on after his death he would have been so proud of and we all would have loved Dad to be around, as well; seeing the grandchildren. Jenna, I know, he would have been so proud of. I miss the competing, especially with Rocco in the crowd pulling for me. The batting practice I still throw to the college kids and Legion kids is still fun. But, I don't like anyone hitting me so I still like it but not the part of laying it in there for the hitters to hit. They don't understand.

I hear Kenny Mazonson at times telling the kids "In Dave's day, you wouldn't be able to even make contact with him." I still think of that as the "pride" factor. I had way too much pride to be just a good pitcher. You have to have the "you know what" to get on that mound. You can't give someone a set of balls. They either have them or they don't. You can't tell someone some day "Oh, you're tough today." It just won't happen. Too many people walk around with suits on and they think they're tough. I used to wear a suit to work every day and I was known as a regular guy, but the guys knew I was, if they put me in that position. I would drive places with my old boss and he would get mouthy when he was with me. I knew he couldn't fend for himself. But that was the coward in him; no courage. But that's what part of my life is all about. Pride and doing things the right way. I can be honest. I made a lot of mistakes along the way but each mistake was a lesson learned and I tried not to make it again. I lived a great life that most people would love to have lived even with the detours that came with it. I persevered and beat the odds. I always wanted that one person to say I couldn't do something so that I could prove them wrong. I have a wonderful family and friends everywhere.

Roseann and I haven't been seeing each other of late. But we know we are still friends and she's a great girl. That's the Caiazzo genes in me. Always looking for the one that I know is going to be the one person that I have the most trust and confidence in. The one that will catch my attention with the qualities in a person I'm looking for will be the one. Over the years there have been so many but I always have my doubts and I want that one special person to be the only one.

An old high school teammate of mine came down to one of our Legion baseball games that I coach. His name is Joe Levine. He came by the dugout and, after a hard-hit grounder was fielded nicely by our second baseman,, he said, "Cai, could you still have caught that ball now?" I answered, "No." He responded, "Only because you wouldn't allow anyone to harm that handsome face." People over the years would tease me all the time by kind of shadowing the saying that they used to say about Joe Pep. They'd say, "Davey Cai would have it no other way."

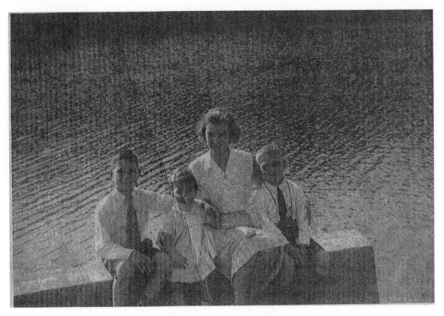

Steve, Joan, Mom and Dave in the early years

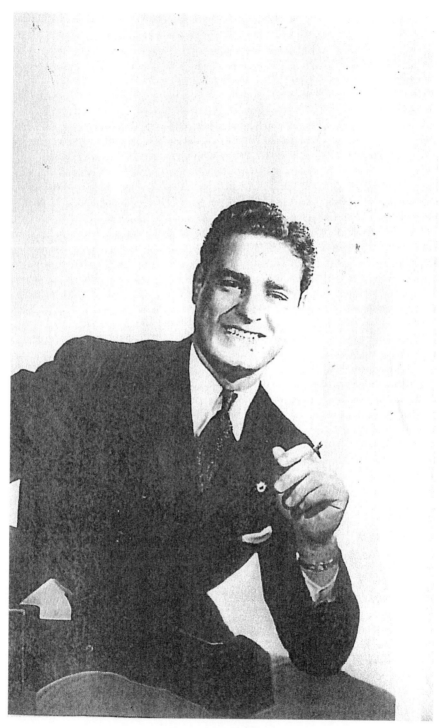

Rocco in Hollywood

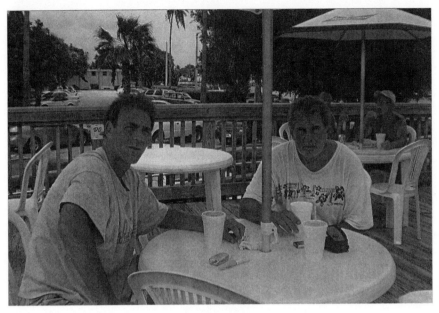

Dave and his brother, Steve, in Ft. Myers Beach

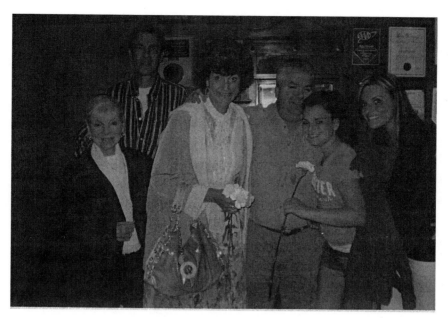

Mom, Dave, Joan, Jack, Melissa and Bethann during the holidays

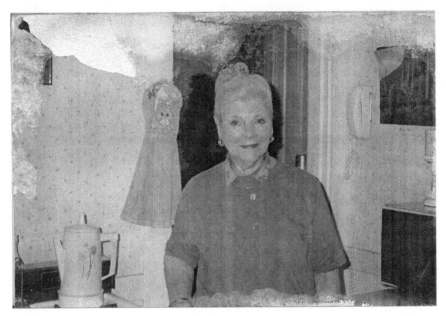

Angelina Caiazzo

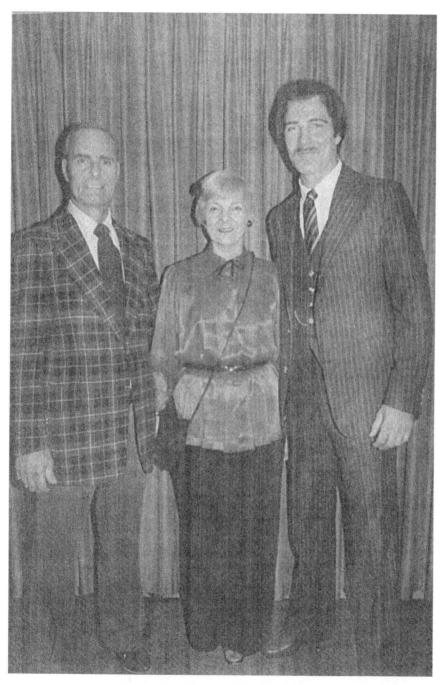

Rocco, Angelina and Dave at a banquet

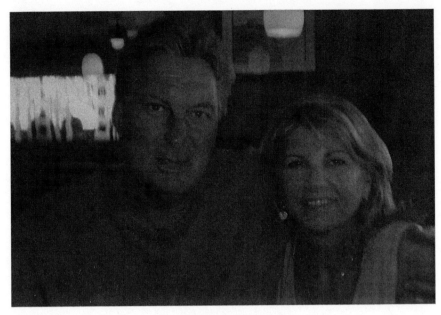

Steve and Susan

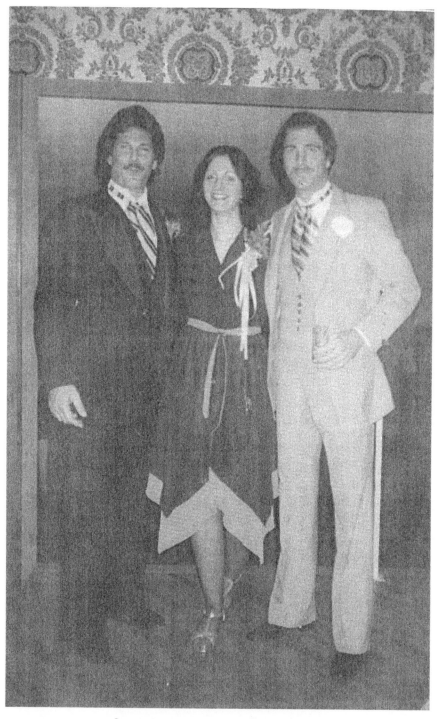

Steve, Joan and Dave at Steve's wedding

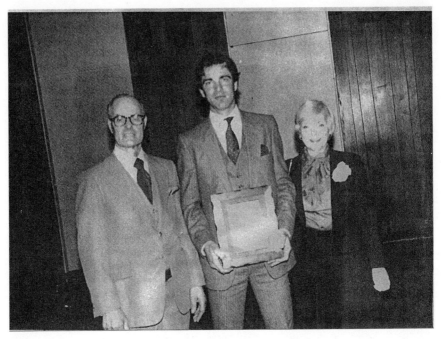

Dad, Dave and Mom at a banquet

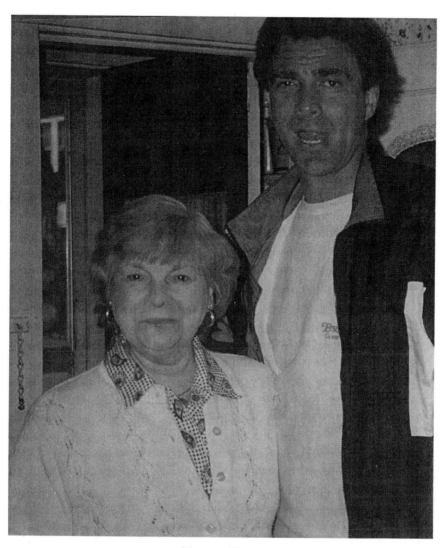

Mom and Dave

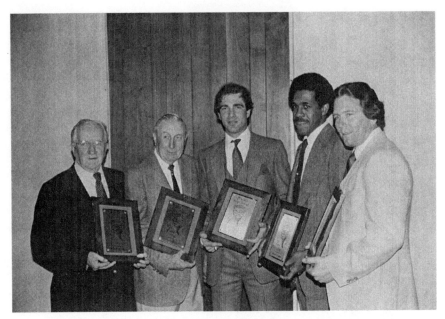

Malden High School's first Hall of Fame banquet. Inductees, from left,
Eddie Melanson, Charlie O'Rourke, Dave, Willie Barron and John Salmon

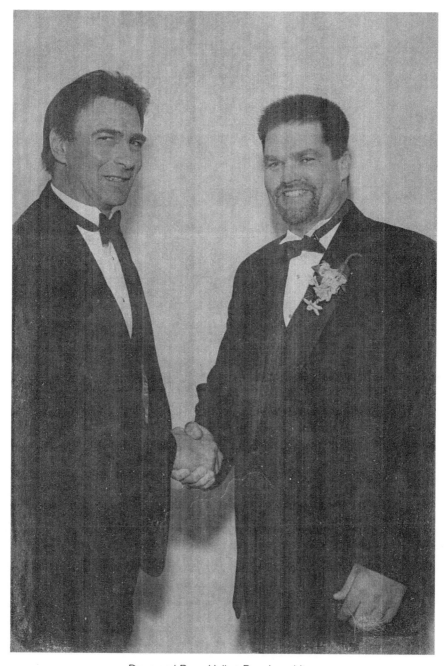

Dave and Russ Hall at Russ' wedding

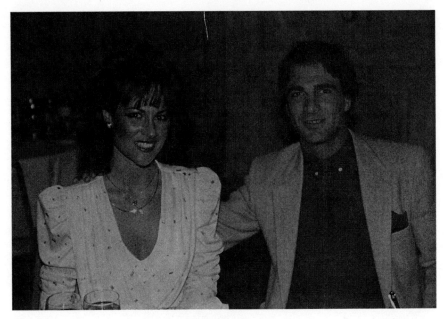

Janet and Dave

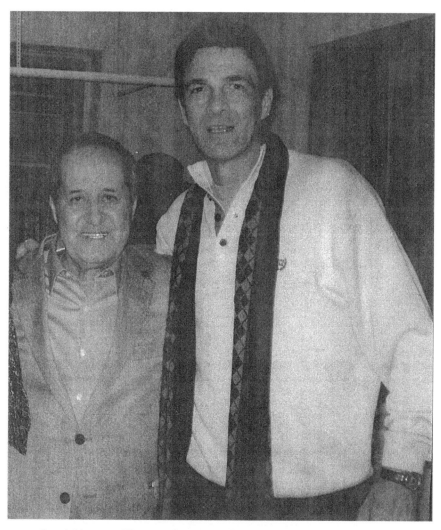

Coach Vieira and Dave at Coach's uniform number retirement ceremony

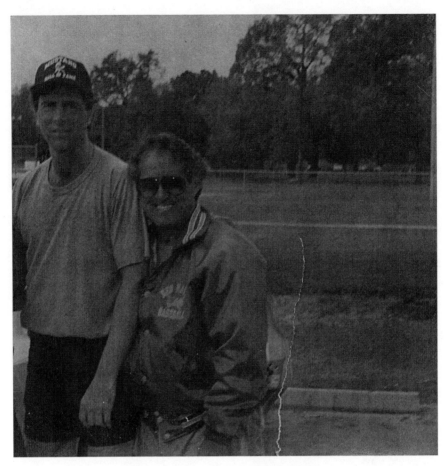

Dave and Coach V in Ormond, Florida

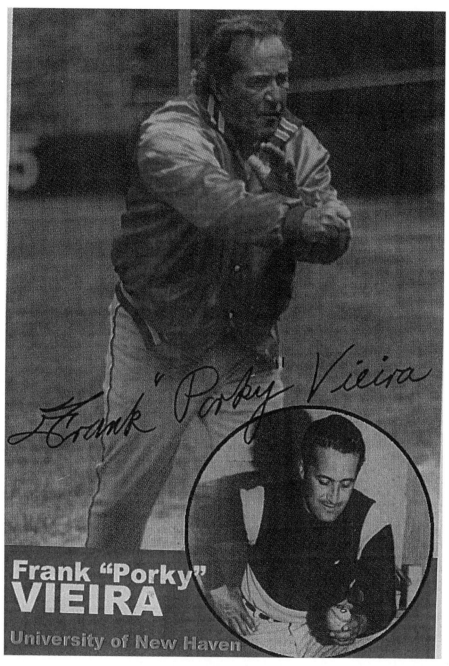

Coach V showing his style of coaching

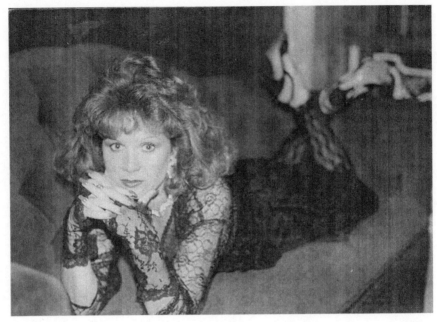

Melinda

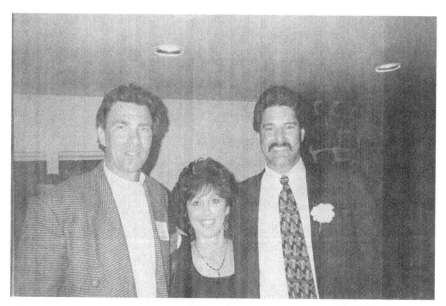

Dave and Cy Young Award winner Steve Bedrosian with Betsy at the University of New Haven Hall of Fame

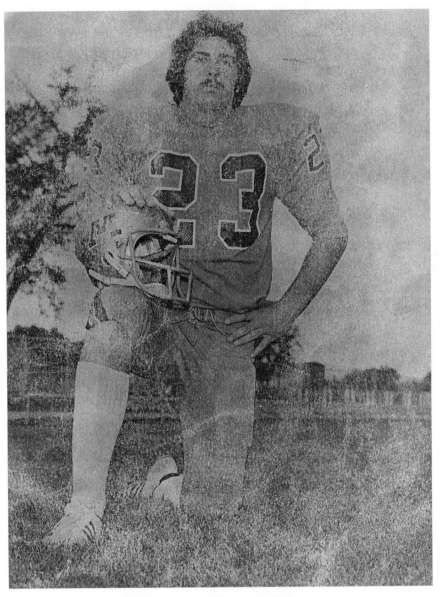

Steve Caiazzo at the University of Minnesota

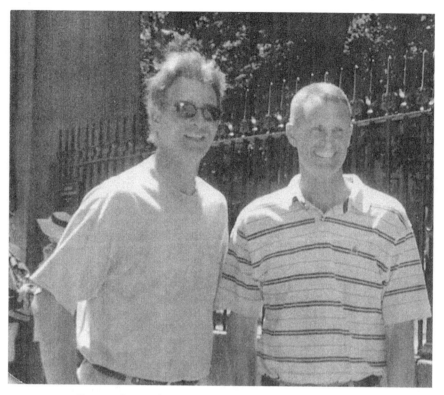

Dave and minor league teammate and catcher Fla Strawn

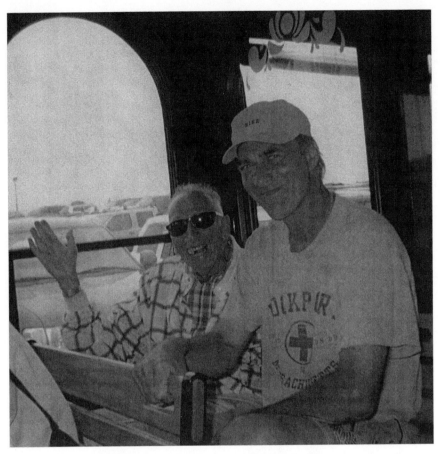

Ralph Myerow and Dave in York Beach, Maine

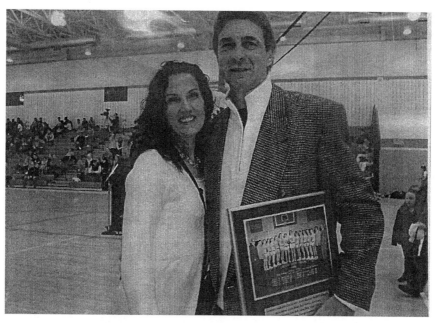

Roseann and Dave at the New Haven banquet

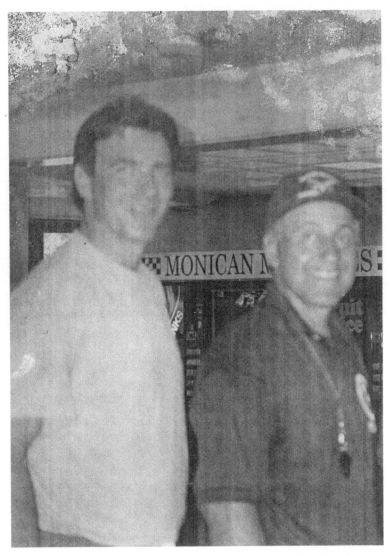

Dave and former Red Sox star Rico Petrocelli, a great friend

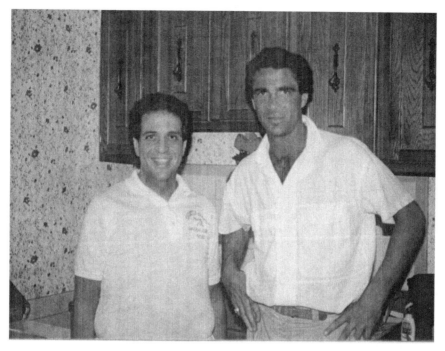

Long-time friend John "Trixie" Trischitta and Dave

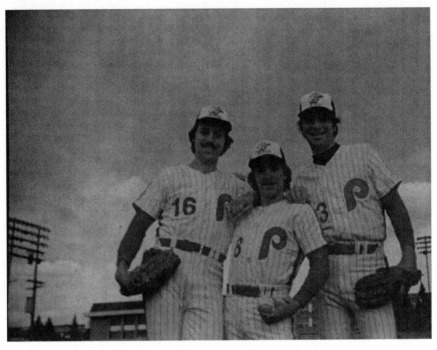

Ralph Suarez and Paco Jonis with Dave in Butte, Montana

Perspectives on Dave Caiazzo

Frank Adorn

Dave's coach at Malden High

"Dave just loved baseball. He was very serious about the sport. Whatever we instructed, Dave carried it out. He absorbed everything. He still loves the game.

"Obviously, Dave was one of the best players I coached, one of the best I ever saw. Whenever he took the mound, we were confident that we were going to win the game."

Russ Hall

Dave's friend since high school

"I first saw Dave in a Babe Ruth League (practice game) in 1968. A teammate of mine and someone that played with Dave in junior high was Hank O'Brien. The conversation went like this:

Hank: 'What do you think of the pitcher on the mound now?'

Me: 'Wow, he's big for a 15-year-old.'

Hank: 'Actually, he is only 13 and is already the best pitcher in the league.'

"I remember at 13, I was probably 5 ft. 4 in. and was looking at some-one my age that was probably 6 ft. 2 in. at the time. I remember thinking 'damn, what do they feed these kids on the west side of the city.'

"The next year we met in high school in tenth-grade science class and eventually started hanging around in 1970 with John Lopresti. My initial impression was that Dave was a good guy and most definitely a baseball junkie. He knew the stances of many major league players and pitching motions, as well. We would play stickball games in his driveway with his brother Steve and his friend Doug, aka Superman. Dave would bat from both sides of the plate, again copying almost perfectly the stances and swings of his favorite team, the Yankees.

"Dave had gotten diabetes just a short time before I really knew him. I did not really know what it was at that time. He was the first person I actu-ally met that had this disease. I know that I had a great grandmother who lost her leg because of this disease. However, I had never met her and it did not really impact me that much. In later years, I realized what a debilitating disease it is.

"Baseballwise, it did not seem to affect Dave's performance. He was head and shoulders above everybody else. I learned later on that it clearly did have an effect on him and he just concealed it. He would bring orange juice and other quick fixes for sugar that would boost his blood sugar count and get him through a game.

"One thing we joke about was the American Legion tryouts were tak-ing place at Devir Park. While Dave already had a secured spot on the team, I, as usual, was on the brink. There were 19 guys left with only 18 roster spots. I threw the last inning of a scrimmage game and loaded the bases with two out. Dave steps up to the plate and the first pitch, boom, long fly ball over the center fielder's head. Grand slam. I was informed about fifteen minutes later that I was cut. Good friend, hmmmm!!

"The first time we were on a team together was our senior year. Con-sidering, I was not a very athletic guy, I felt fortunate to have made the var-sity. Sometimes being solidified on the bench you do become observant. An article in one of the Malden papers suggested that if Malden had nine Dave Caiazzos, they would have the best pitching, fielding and hitting in the GBL, which was pretty much the same view as I had.

"My favorite game that Dave pitched in high school was against North Quincy at Devir Park. There was a rumor that there were going to be a lot of scouts at the game to watch Dave. There was a group of them behind the screen but Dave gave up three runs in the first inning and all but two of them left. He wasn't pitching well and the three runs seemed insurmountable but Dave came back and threw shutout ball the rest of the game and we won 8-3. I believe Dave hit a home run and drove in most of the runs. That showed how determined he is as a pitcher. He channeled his anger when he pitched. Dave had a nasty side to himself when he pitched. He wanted to be the best; he was ultra competitive.

"Obviously the stats support Dave's 20-strikeout Everett game as his very best game. I also remember the Sandlot All-Star game at Fenway. Dave was selected to that team and I knew that his arm was really hurting him. He did however pitch well and faced the minimum amount of batters without allowing a hit or walk. This was probably the beginning period where arm problems would start to become more of an issue later on.

"It was in junior college that Dave kind of groomed himself for a bigger college career. There were many good players on these Mo Maloney-coached teams: DJ Saulnier, John Greeley and John Valeri to name a few.

"I once asked Dave when he felt he threw the hardest. He said, 'I would probably say Mass. Bay.' The reason I asked was because I used to catch him down the park all the time. Definitely not on the top of my list of favorite things to do. My hand would be red and swollen, by the time he would be done (probably about 100 pitches). At the end he wanted to simulate game conditions for an inning. That meant three make believe hitters. Well, I would pretty much call nine consecutive strikes. My hand was sore and I just wanted to get the hell out of there. He once got Jim Carey to catch him one day. Jim was not a baseball guy. Dave threw him a curveball that landed in the dirt about a foot before the plate. It bounced up and hit him right in gonads! Ouch!

"I went down to a game in Franklin, Mass., where Dave was pitching in a regional tournament game against Dean Junior College. I got lost and did not make it there until about the eighth inning. Mass. Bay lost. I believe it was a 1-0 game. Dave looked at me after the game was over. No acknowledgement, just an icy stare. He walked by me went to his car and probably did not talk to anyone for a few days. That was his competitive nature. No doubt, he had a temper and pitched with that same nasty intensity. He pitched with a chip on his shoulder and it definitely showed.

"One thing that helped Dave was his older brother, Steve, who had gone through all the same things Dave was going through. Steve graduated two years earlier. He was a terrific athlete and no doubt was a big influence on Dave, his career and his approach to baseball. Steve was dominant in football, starred at a junior college in Nebraska and went on to play for Minnesota in the Big 10. There were a lot of parallels in their athletic careers. Steve would always push Dave, not giving a lot of credit when he pitched well. He always told him that he could always do better whether it meant throwing harder, striking out more hitters, hit with more power, etc. I believe that it made Dave a tough, hard-nosed pitcher who always wanted to win the battle, no matter what the situation was. Steve was forceful and I believe was Dave's biggest and best role model.

"Dave also got a lot of that mental toughness from his father. He was a great guy who gave everything he had to his family.

The trip to New York with Steve Ring, Dave and myself

"Dave asked me to go with Steve Ring and him to a San Francisco-Mets game because Steve Bedrosian, former New Haven pitcher and friend of Dave's, was then with the Giants. I asked him who was going to drive. He told me that he would. At the time he had a small sports car, a Nissan 200sx that was big enough for two people in the front seat and a small dog in the back. I told Dave, no way am I going to sit in that back seat to and from New York. He said, 'Steve will take the back seat on the way home.' I said, 'Stevie with his ego in the back seat of a small car like this, no way!' I suggested we take my car so I drove both ways. At least I had the front seat. We stopped first in Manhattan and went to Mickey Mantle's place, then made our way towards Shea Stadium. I took the George Washington Bridge and got in a lane that did not have a toll booth collector. Not wanting to risk getting pulled over by the police, I then parked and started jumping from toll booth to toll booth and finally paid the $2.50 fee. When I got back to the car, they (Steve and Dave) were in hysterics. They said I looked like OJ (before) when he ran through the airport terminals in the Hertz commercials. I got the last laugh however. We went to the hotel that Bedrosian was in. He had not arrived so we went to a nearby pub. Will Clark was in line. Steve said, 'I coached him down the Cape. He will remember me.' So he went over and said 'I coached you in the Cape Cod League All Star game.' Clark did not recall this. He kept asking him questions about Bedrosian and when would he be arriving. Finally, Clark said tersely, 'Listen buddy, it's not my day to watch him!' and then went to be seated. Bedrosian left us some guest passes, and then we tried to get down near the dugout and had an usher to contend with. Steve was telling the usher how he had coached a lot of these guys down the Cape League. However, I do not believe the usher was buying it. Steve, while still embarrassed from the pub incident and now the usher (Steve was telling the truth as he had been a long-time

Harwich Mariners coach), finally got his wish and he and Dave went down to the Giants dugout. I stayed behind and watched from an exit in an area so far away binoculars would not have done any good.

The ULowell game after Dave had graduated (early '90s)

"This was the game Dave and I were supposed to go to and see a 19-0 New Haven team face UMass Lowell. Dave couldn't make it due to work, so I went by myself. Dave asked me to stop at Dunkin' Donuts and get Coach V some chocolate chip cookies because he loves them before a game. Well, I get to the park and speak to one of his players near the dugout. I asked for Coach V and told him that I was a friend of Cai's. Coach V was expecting Dave and came out of the dugout. First thing he says is 'where is Cai?' I said he had to work. I then gave him the cookies and his reply was a sarcastic 'gee, thanks!' I watched the game by the side of the dugout. New Haven dropped two and scored one run in two games dropping them to 19-2. Coach later called Dave and said, 'That jinx bastard son of a bitch comes to the game dressed completely in black. I need base hits and this son of a bitch brings me cookies. What the freak. Cai, tell that jinx S.O.B. to stay away from our games.' In later years I would bring him a bottle of vodka and he told Cai that I was a good soul. He actually preferred to just get the bottle and then not take the chance of having me at the game.

Best purpose pitch

"No doubt, I witnessed this one first hand. Malden Square in the early 1970s. A person I will call Chucky (not his real name as I do not want to embarrass him), was having a verbal joust with Dave and it got a little heated. The next thing I knew, Dave fired a fastball, not with a baseball, but a large Italian sub, right square off the kisser of Chucky. Here he was with pickles, tomatoes, onions and oil dripping from his forehead. Wow, talk about backing someone off the plate!

Dave the umpire

"This was truly classic. If you never saw Dave umpire, you really missed something. What a show! Typically, it would go something like this with Dave behind the plate and a coach questioning his calls.

Coach : 'C'mon blue (after a low pitch was called a strike), pick it up will ya.'

At this point, Dave would just look over at the bench, although I knew he was starting to get pissed. Then would come strike two, basically for the coach.

Coach: 'C'mon blue, be consistent. My god you have been all over the place.'

Now, I know Dave does not like to be questioned about anything with baseball, so with that, he would flip off the mask and tell the coach to shut up if he wants to remain on the bench.

Next the proverbial strike three.

Coach: 'Another lousy call, blue, you are going to cost us the game.' Dave now throws the mask off and the chest guard down and walks toward the bench to confront the coach

Dave: 'I am going to cost you the game? Are you shitting me? Your team can't hit, can't pitch and you are a terrible coach. By the way where did you play ball? Yeah right, you didn't, just as I thought. Just sit down, shut up and I don't want to hear another word out of you.' Silence for the rest of the game.

"Dave was known for his temper, but the most classic line I ever heard about it was from a doorman at the Copley Plaza (named Jimmy). It went like this: 'I really like Dave, he is a great guy, but the one thing about him is he doesn't have a temper. OK, so he is still looking to get even with the doctor that slapped him when he was born, but other than that...' Classic.

Diabetes and the day-to-day dealings with it

"Dave got the disease at a young age. He has gone through different stages dealing with and trying to manage this disease. When we were younger, he did not want anyone to even broach the subject. In some ways, I believe he looked at it as a sign of weakness. So, when I could see that he was starting to get low, I would generally try and get him something to eat or drink, but kind of in a subtle way. I learned quite a bit about how it can impact a person. Sluggishness, chronic fatigue, moodiness, temporary inability to process thoughts and obviously things much worse. Dave probably was in his early 30s when he stopped trying to hide it and became more open as to how it affected him.

"Often times, I would see that he would have about a 10-minute window to get something in his system, when his sugar levels dropped. If he did not get food or something to drink in that time frame, he would often times have a hard time conveying his thoughts. When he would finally get something into his system, it would probably take about thirty to forty-five minutes to get back to normal. You could see how fatigued it left him. I am sure it just shocks the whole body. He once told me 'I cannot remember one single day since I got diabetes that I did not feel tired.'

"One day, I mentioned to him an incident about someone I knew (a woman whose husband had diabetes). Her husband got killed in a motor vehicle accident while driving on the wrong side of the highway, after passing out at the wheel of the car while having a diabetic reaction. I will never forget his response. After pondering what had happened, he told me 'that will probably happen to me someday.' I did not know what to say, but I believe that it was really the way he felt. Got to be an awful hard thing to live with.

On Dave's father

"Truly one of the nicest guys I have ever met. He would certainly do anything for anybody. In many ways, he was a father figure to me, a person I could relate to. He was an instinctive person who watched things closely and took it all in. I believe the three most influential people that Dave had were his father, his brother and Coach Vieira. When Dave's father passed away in 1988, it was an especially sad day for me. Dave gave a really nice tribute to his father at the New Haven Hall of Fame banquet."

Coach V (Frank "Porky" Vieira)

Dave's coach at New Haven

"Dave Caiazzo was the most courageous player I coached in all my time (44 years) at New Haven. Despite the diabetes, he performed. He took us to the World Series. Really, the only time he ever lost was when I overused him. How he got through all those years pitching with diabetes I don't know.

"One of the games that really stands out the most came when our backs were up against the wall and we had to beat LeMoyne to get to the College World Series. He and I were riding down in the elevator to get ready to go to the game. I asked him if he was ready. Dave said, 'I'll handle it,' and he did. We won the game and played in the World Series.

"It's funny. When I went to scout Dave before he came to New Haven, in the game I saw he stunk out the place but I liked the way he reacted when he got beat. There was something, the look on his face, that said he was a real competitor. When the money was on the line, Dave was the best.

"Because of the diabetes, we had orange juice and chocolate in the dugout for him. Even when he wasn't feeling his best, Dave would fight through it. He was tough as nails.

"As a person, there is not enough you can say about Dave. He is the most warm-hearted guy I've ever known. He still calls me once a week even now. I have never heard anyone say a bad word about him. Everything he does is positive."

Steve Caiazzo

Dave's brother

"Even though I'm a bit older, Dave was always one step ahead of me. He's a lot more organized than I am. He always had things lined up and written out on small pieces of paper. He had everything down as to what he was doing that day. He was fully prepared and that carried over into his pitching. However, as the older brother, I used to chase him around the yard and up the stairs. I was kind of the tough guy.

"Dave was all baseball. He lived it, ate it and drank it. It was strictly baseball with him and baseball has given him an endless number of friends.

"We both set our sights very high. As a kid, I'd be watching Ohio State football on TV and I said 'I want to play there.' Dave was the same with baseball. He wanted to be a professional baseball player. I played football in the Big Ten and he signed a pro baseball contract.

"Back then, we would go down to the park at 7 a.m. and come home at 8 p.m. There would be 12 to 15 kids show up. Sometimes we'd play wiffle ball. We had a home plate and a pitcher's mound made of plaster of Paris. Dave and I would go back and forth in those games. My guy back then was Willie Mays and his guy was Mickey Mantle. I'd be jabbering at him and then I'd chase him into the house.

"When Dave was a sophomore at Malden High, I was a senior and we both played on the varsity. He really came into his own as a junior. That was when he showed he could pitch against older players. Both pitching and hitting, he was dominant. That was when he started to develop a slider and a good curve. Dave could place them and his fastball where he wanted. He was striking out 15, 18 batters a game. Then he played at Mass. Bay and really stepped it up when he was at the University of New Haven.

"Honestly, Dave can be thick-headed. I can say that because I'm his brother. He just doesn't like to be criticized. We butted heads over many things over the years but he's my brother and I really care about him."

John "Trixie" Trischitta

Dave's long-time friend

"Dave's calling in life is baseball. For him, pitching is an art. Dave can watch someone throw one or two pitches and he can see anything that needs to be corrected. He had his baseball camp for years, he gives pitching lessons and he has helped coach a number of teams, high school, college and Legion but he's never been a head coach. Any team that had Dave as a head coach would benefit greatly. To some degree, I think maybe he missed his calling.

"Dave kept getting better and better, through high school, at Mass. Bay and then at New Haven. His senior year at New Haven, I saw most of his games, even the Southern trips. He was already having some arm problems then but he was nearly unhittable.

"Most of the years he was in the Intercity League, I was with another team. There were many pitchers in the league who could throw hard but Dave could do that and put the ball exactly where he wanted it. During that time, he always had to overcome the diabetes and a sore arm. You would hear some guys talk about having a sore arm and use it as an excuse. Dave never used his disability as a crutch and he never said anything about his arm problem.

On the cruise

"We went on a cruise one time and were really enjoying ourselves. We became friends with a bunch of girls. It was great. Then Dave had a diabetic attack. That night he started talking ridiculous. We went out on the deck and he got a burger. He was in a chaise lounge and the plate started to slip off his stomach. I grabbed it and he got mad. Then the dish hit the floor. I looked and Dave was foaming at the mouth. It was really scary. They got a stretcher and rushed him to the infirmary. It took a long time for Dave to recover from that. To this day, when we go out to eat, he's says, 'Remind me to take my needle.'

At Steve Bedrosian's wedding

"Dave became good friends with Steve Bedrosian (former Cy Young Award winner with the Phillies in 1987). Steve was a few years behind Dave at New Haven and Dave was helping out with the team when Bedrock was there. Bedrosian always credited Dave for playing a key role in his pitching development. We got invited to Bedrosian's wedding in South Carolina. Dave always left the travelling details to me. We flew into Charlotte and then we had to take another flight to Spartanburg. I made a mistake on the departure time. When I realized it, we got into a cab and told the driver to go as fast as he could. We just made it through the security check in time and we got on the plane just as they were closing the door. We did have a great time at the wedding."

Italian baseball

"At one time, it looked as though Dave was going to play professional baseball in Italy. There was a rule in that league that a parent had to be an Italian citizen when the player was born. Dave's father was born in Italy but he had become an American citizen by the time Dave was born. That was holding things up. Then Dave got a call that he had to be at the Italian consulate in New York City as soon as possible. We were in Daytona Beach with a couple of girls. We got up at 5 a.m. and got on a plane to fly to New York. Then we got to New Haven to pick up Coach V and his wife and we had to drive back to New York, where we were going to stay in his cousin Nick's apartment. Nick was going out on the town at about 11 p.m. and we went out with him. By the time we got back, it was 5 a.m. and Dave had to be at the consulate at 10 a.m. The night before, Nick had said he wanted to go with us but I was snoring so loud that he didn't get any sleep, so he just rolled over and stayed in the apartment. Dave went to the consulate and then we went back to New Haven by car. After all that, he never played in Italy."

Pro tryout

"When it looked like Dave was going to get a chance to sign, Coach V arranged a tryout where Dave was going to throw batting practice for New Haven in the Yale Bowl. While he warming up, Coach V said to the scouts that one of the best things about Dave's pitching is his control. The New Haven kids were supposed to rotate in and out of the batting cage for Dave but then he hit the first one, and then he hit another. Pretty soon, the New Haven players were all standing outside the batting cage.

"Despite that, they signed Dave to a contract where he was going to Montana to report June 15 and play through the end of August. They offered him two deals, $500 a month and they would pay his airfare or $600 and he would play his own way. At first, he took the $600 deal but then we looked into how much it would cost to fly to Butte, Montana. Dave renegotiated right away."

Steve Ring

Former coach, long-time friend

"Dave is a one-in-a-million guy and I say that from my heart. I've known Dave for four decades as a person and as an athlete. I was an assistant coach at Malden High when Dave was a sophomore and he caught my eye right away because he had so much determination and intensity as a pitcher. When he saw a batter digging in against him, Dave would put him on his rear. I followed Dave's growth and it was by leaps and bounds, gaining complete command of the strike zone. He was a tall beanpole who became a mature, professional person. He reminded me of Jim Palmer. When Dave was on the mound it was like having an extra coach on the field.

"Truly, if it was the seventh game of the World Series or the deciding game in the Cape Cod League, he's the guy I'd want out there. He is at the top of the list for the guys I'd want on the mound. With Dave, you got everything he had in the gas tank. I coached twenty-two guys who made it to the majors and no one gave more effort than Dave.

"He is a disciple of the game. For four decades, in high school, college, in the pros, scouting, running his camp, giving pitching lessons, he has been a great ambassador for baseball.

"Dave and I have had a lot of fun together. When we talk about the old times, the kid in us comes back. One incident was when Dave and Russ Hall and I went to a game at Shea Stadium. After the game we were walking to Mickey Mantle's place. Russ is maybe 6 ft. 4 in., Dave is 6 ft. 5 in. and I'm about 6 ft. 2 in. We were near the Plaza Hotel when a guy comes along the sidewalk and says to me, the smallest, 'I know you. You play for the New York Giants.' We laugh about that every time we mention it.

"My wife, Donna, and I had met about four or five of Dave's girl-friends. We were visiting Dave at his townhouse and he invited us up. On the stairway was a photo of a girl and Donna blurts out, 'I never met her. Where did she come from?' That was Dave and his current girlfriend.

"When we were younger, Dave, Trixie, Carl and I were up at Amerige Park. I was wearing glasses and Carl was making some comments. Carl got to the point with me where I had had it. I gave my glasses to Dave and was going to kill Carl but he took off running all around Amerige Park with everyone laughing.

"I am proud and happy to have Dave as a friend. I consider him, truly, my best friend, and just a great human being."

Ken Mazonson

Friend, coach and fellow diabetic

"I have known Dave since high school but our friendship really didn't strike up until years later. We had the obvious similarity in loving baseball. A mutual friend contacted Dave and then Dave called me and offered me a spot working in his camp and I worked there for fifteen or more years.

"Our friendship certainly evolved from baseball. We are on the same page about the sport. We're two old-time baseball junkies. We're sort of hard-liners when it comes to the sport. We always subscribe to the same principles. I asked Dave to help me coach the Legion team in Malden five years ago. We'll be at practices or at games and throwing around the same thoughts.

"Then there's the diabetes. We both have been diabetic pretty much all our lives. We have had that in common since we were young. I sort of watch over him. There was one time after a day at his camp when I followed him home to make sure he made it. Another time, we were wrapping up the camp and he kept repeating himself. We got in touch with a Malden Police officer whose son was at the camp and she made sure Dave got home OK.

"Then there was the time I got a call from a mother who wanted Dave to give her son pitching lessons. She kept calling him and got no answer. She knew I lived close to Dave so she called. I ran down to Dave's house. I don't know how he even opened the door. He was really out of it. He had dropped a glass on the floor and it broke. Dave must have passed out and then came to. I couldn't remember him ever being like that but he did get through it.

"Dave is the most competitive perfectionist I've ever been around. With the Legion team, we could have a pitcher strike out ten batters but Dave will want to know why he walked two. And I've heard him ask other people where they have played baseball and at what level whenever they say something about the game.

"There is another story about the camp. Dave would have an instructor be the administrator of the camp. It was a lot of work doing all the registering, collecting the money, scheduling, ordering everything. It seemed that after two years, Dave would get another administrator. I was at the camp twelve or fourteen years and went through seven administrators. Every one of them would come up to me and ask what the discounts were all about. Those of us who had been there a few years would say, 'Dave's going out with another kid's mother.' It became a standing joke."

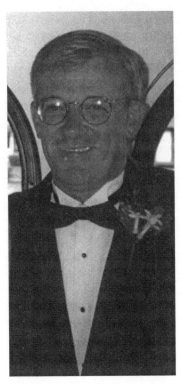

Paul Leahy was the sports editor of the Malden Evening News for more than twenty years. He is a graduate of Arlington Catholic High School (where his only athletic claim to fame is scoring the school's first touchdown) and Northeastern University. Paul and his wife Anne have three children, Eirinn, Tim and Eileen, and are the proud grandparents of Emily and Drew. Paul works in the Athletic Department at Regis College and spends too much time playing golf on Cape Cod. Paul met Dave Caiazzo when Dave was a star pitcher for Malden High School. Paul followed and wrote about Dave's career as it progressed from American Legion ball, to Mass. Bay Community College, to the University of New Haven, to the pro ranks and during two stints in the Intercity League, where Dave was the dominant pitcher for the better part of a decade. They have remained friends for more than four decades and when they get together, somehow the conversation usually starts and ends with baseball.